HOW TO STAY S[ANE IN AN] INSANE WORLD

To Roja

May my book bring you peace of mind.

By T. Riojas

T. Riojas

Woodbridge Publishers

1280 Lexington Ave STE 2

New York, NY 10028

Copyright © 2024 T. Riojas
All rights reserved

First Edition

ISBN (Paperback):978-1-917184-03-8

ISBN (Hardback):978-1-917184-04-5

No part of this publication may be reproduced, stored in a retrieval system, copied in any form or by any means, electronic, mechanical, photocopying, recording or otherwise transmitted without written permission from the publisher. You must not circulate this book in any format.

Under no circumstances will any blame or legal responsibility be held against the publisher, or author, for any damages, reparation, or monetary loss due to the information contained within this book, either directly or indirectly.

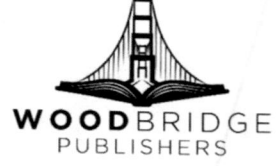

WOODBRIDGE
PUBLISHERS

TABLE OF CONTENTS

Chapter 1: Understanding Fear 1
   The Mental Projection of Fear..1
Chapter 2: Self Care 5
   What is pampering?..5
   What is faith?...6
Chapter 3: Building Healthy Relationship 8
   Character of Healthy and Unhealthy Relationship 8
   Healthy Relationship 9
   How to achieve a healthy Relationship?.......................11
      Declare your Independence 12
      Rise and Shine...13
      Set Boundaries 14
      Date Yourself...14
Chapter 4: Financial Wellness 16
   Develop a Budget 17
   Contacting Creditors 18
   Credit Counseling..19
   Auto and Home Loans 21
   Debt Consolidation 22
   Bankruptcy..24
Chapter 5: What Does A Boundary Look Like? 27

Invisible Property Lines and Responsibility...........................27
Me and Not Me: Understanding Boundaries.........................28
To and For: Understanding Responsibility 29
Good In, Bad Out: Boundaries For Protection 30
God and Boundaries: Embracing Divine Example 32
Examples of Boundaries 33
    Skin 33
    Words 33
    Truth 34
    Geographical Distance 34
    Time 35
    Emotional Distance 36
    Other People 36
    Consequences 37
What's Within My Boundaries? 38
    Feelings 40
    Attitudes and Beliefs 41
    Behaviors 41
    Choices 42
    Values 43
    Limits 44
    Talents 44
    Thoughts 45
    Desires 46
    Love 48
Boundary Problems 49

Compliant: Saying Yes to the Bad 49

Avoidants: Saying No to the good 50

Controllers: Not Respecting Others' Boundaries 52

Chapter 6: Seek Clarity 55

The Top 3% 56

You're in Good Company 57

A Goal is Like a Destination 58

Step 1: Limit Your Goals to 7-10 59

Step Two: Turn Your Goals Into Vision 63

Step 4: Get Results 65

Step 5: Get Rest 68

Chapter 7: THE POWER OF HAPPINESS 72

Happiness Habit 1: Define & Feel What Happiness Looks Like To YOU 72

Happiness Habit 2: Befriend Your Present 73

Happiness Habit 3: Free Yourself From Overthinking 74

Happiness Habit 4: Focus on A Positive Outcome 75

Happiness Habit 5: Let Go of Specific Outcomes 78

Happiness Habit 6: Don't Be Afraid To Fail 80

Happiness Habit 7: Let Go Of Grudges 80

Happiness Habit 8: Be Grateful For What's in Front of You 81

Happiness Habit #9: Don't Settle For Good Enough 82

Happiness Habit #10: Be Part of Something Bigger 82

Chapter 8: The Quick Hacks To Success 84

Take Creative Time Daily 84

Observe Other Jobs For Gratitude 85

Setting Gratitude Alarms 85
Stash Cash 87
Spoil Yourself Randomly 88
Invest in Yourself 89
Draw Energy From Your Frequent Smiles 89
Find The Good In The Bad 90
Bounce Back Fast 90
Think Solution, Not Problem 91
Ask Happy People 91
Go To Your Happy Place 92
Live Long & Prosper 92
Take Time To Understand 94
Don't Judge 95
Help Those Who Are Worse Off Than You 97
Do Your Best Always 98

Chapter 9: HAVE AN ABUNDANT MINDSET 103
BARELY ENOUGH, JUST ENOUGH AND MORE THAN ENOUGH 104
SKINNY GOAT OR FATTED CALF 105
One Touch of God's Favor 107
A Place of ABUNDANCE 108
Pressed Down and Running Over 109
Out of Lack, Into a Good & Spacious Land 111
The Power To Get Wealth 112
A Thousand Times More 114

About the Author 116

CHAPTER 1: UNDERSTANDING FEAR

The Mental Projection of Fear

While many individuals in our lives might seek to stoke our doubts and fears, the vast majority will seek to support us. More will seek to pull us up than push us down.

People understand that by allowing us to chase our dreams unencumbered, they are silently granting themselves permission to pursue their own.

No matter how many bores and bastards we encounter in life, we must remember that we have friends all around, and we mustn't hesitate to ask for their help, inspiration, and wisdom.

The harsh truth of life is that though fear is often socially cued and conditioned, it more often stems from the neglect of our own minds. We misuse our mental faculties by scarcely using them at all.

We possess the means to extinguish our fears, but we lack the discipline to employ them, akin to having an extinguisher in our hands as our home burns but choosing not to use it because we'd have to aim.

How frequently do we sense worry but, instead of combatting it with conscious thought, allow it to consume us? How often do we fixate on negative thoughts that burgeon into a raging fire of anxiety?

For many, this has occurred unchecked for so long that they are no longer conscious of the predictable thought patterns—all of which they can anticipate, control, and transform—that are causing their fear. They simply feel afraid all the time and believe there is nothing they can do about it, much like the sad child holding a burst balloon she herself popped.

Let us now, once and for all, learn to anticipate how our minds cultivate fear.

Shall we continue thinking negatively? What good will come from focusing on all the loss and hardship we might experience in life? There is no self-awareness in letting fear reign because of own mental sloth. We have the personal power to wield our thoughts will free us or destroy us. Maturity comes in understanding that it is our choice alone to move toward freedom.

Just as we can expect the worriers, weaklings, and wicked to derail us if we are not cautious, we can prepare for how our minds will tear us from happiness and progress.

Most of the fear we feel in life is simply anxiety arising from our anticipation of two kinds of pain that change might bring: the pain associated with loss or hardship.

The first type, loss pain, is a thought pattern in which we worry that we will lose something we cherish if we take any given action. If we fear changing jobs, it is because we don't want to lose our compensation, our friendships with certain coworkers, or our corner office. This thought pattern plays out in millions of subtle decisions throughout people's lives.

We think, "If I go on a new diet, I'm afraid I'll lose the joy I feel in eating my favorite foods." "If I quit smoking, I'll lose that 20 minutes of peace I get by going outside and taking long drags, so I am afraid to quit." "If I leave the jerk, I'm afraid I'll lose love in my life and never find anyone else."

The only way to combat this thought pattern is to analyze it closely, then reverse it. Once we sense that we are anticipating loss, we must question whether or not it is true. The more we look for evidence of our fears, the more we realize they are faulty, quick assumptions of a tired or undirected mind. The small, poorly conditioned person may guess that things will be bad, whereas an intelligent, self-aware person may come to a logical conclusion based on real-world evidence or thoughtful principle.

The person who examines their fear of dieting, quitting a bad habit, or leaving a bad relationship comes to realize there is always less to lose than gain in making healthy decisions for themselves. This reframing requires intelligence and optimism.

Once we question the assumption causing us anxiety, we should explore the opposite of our worries, focusing as obsessively as possible on what might be gained if we changed. What if we begin the new diet and find new foods and recipes we love? What if we quit smoking and learn new practices that give us even more relaxation? What if, in a new romantic relationship, we finally find joy? We should certainly visualize these outcomes as much as we visualize dark scenes of loss. Dream up and focus on the positive, for it is much more useful than the long nightmares of negativity.

The second thought pattern that causes us to fear change is related to the anticipation of hardship. We are scared to do something because we think it will be too hard on us. We worry we're not capable or worthy enough to succeed. But isn't it true that with enough time, effort, and dedication, we can learn most of what we need to succeed? Isn't it true that most great accomplishments were achieved by people who, at first, had no idea what they were doing, who had to endure years of struggle to bring their dreams into fruition?

Let's not forget that we didn't always know how to ride a bike or use a computer or make love, but we figured it out. Humans did not know how to land on the moon, but we decided it was a worthwhile endeavor, and so we struggled for a decade to puzzle it out. We became capable of the impossible. Thus is the story of the individual and the entire species. And yet, look how small we let our minds be in so many cases.

We think, "I'm scared to go on a diet because I don't know if I can handle learning new recipes fast enough or endure a 30-minute workout." "I'm afraid of quitting because it will be hard to know what to do with my hands without a cigarette in them." "I'm too freaked out to leave my bad relationship because going online to find someone new sounds like a hassle." We are more than small thoughts.

At some point, maturity will pounce on us and ask, "Are you more than your tiny worries about inconvenience? Isn't a better life worth it?" The only way to break these thought patterns is to question and reverse them. If we simply take a moment to contemplate, we can realize we have learned and endured what is needed; now the tools to manage the difficulties of life are within reach. Perhaps we can imagine ourselves actually enjoying the struggle versus fearing it. We can think, "I'm looking forward to learning to cook new foods." "I'm looking forward to working out with my friends." "I am excited to quit smoking because I can see myself getting up the stairs without being winded and having a life free of addiction." "I'm thrilled to look for someone who is more right for me than my last relationship, to find real love, to enjoy life with my soul mate."

Let us fire our enthusiasm, knowing that the learning journey to freedom can be exciting. We must trust this. We can learn and we can grow, and we must begin now, for destiny favors the bold. To some, this sounds like mere positive thinking, and what of it?

How do you deal with fear? What causes you to fear?

CHAPTER 2: SELF CARE

What is pampering?

Pampering is an inside job, inner grooming, so to speak. It refuels and recharges your mind, body, and spirit, infusing your life with major joy. The focus of pampering is always brought back to the inner self, and in turn, it transforms your outer self. Pampering taps you into the essence of your personal joy, not culturally or socially dictated or determined, but personally defined.

To keep us crystal clear about what qualifies as pampering, I'd like to share three criteria that must be achieved simultaneously—not one or two in isolation from the others—to be considered pampering:

1. **You Are the Primary Beneficiary:** The experience is one in which you are the primary beneficiary. It's intended to be a direct experience where your joy, inner renewal, and peace of mind are the primary objectives. Thus, you being the primary beneficiary is an essential first criterion for pampering. Personal pampering is uniquely for you, not for your man or your friends.

2. **Brings You Joy:** A pampering experience is one that brings you joy, not just happiness. Pampering experiences are joy-focused and joy-centered. This distinction is crucial. Something that "makes you happy" causes you to become pleased, often relying on external factors. However, an experience "that brings joy" goes much deeper, tapping into

a place within yourself that is the source of your joy. It comes from an inside source, not relying on external validation or reasons.

3. **Nurtures Body, Mind, and Spirit:** Pampering nurtures your body, mind, and spirit, increasing your inner peace. The word "nurture" means to nourish, develop, and cultivate. Inner peace is an internal state of serenity and harmonious thoughts and feelings. Pampering should contribute to this sense of inner peace, providing a holistic nourishment for your entire being.

By meeting all three criteria simultaneously, pampering becomes a truly enriching and fulfilling experience, elevating your well-being on multiple levels.

What is faith?

Remember, faith and fear move in opposite directions. Faith is the assurance of things hoped for, the evidence of things not seen. While we often associate faith with religious or theological contexts, we demonstrate faith every day in the routines of our lives.

Consider flying—it takes faith to step into a metal tube and hurtle through the air thirty thousand feet above the ground while traveling at five hundred miles per hour. Every time you board a plane, you are acting on faith in the pilot, just as surely as you can put your faith in Jesus.

Paul tells us that the purpose of the shield of faith is to protect us from all the fiery darts of the wicked one. These darts are as varied as the insidious lies that promote them and include not only temptations to ungodly behavior, doubt, and despair, but also persecution and false teaching.

Faith is belief plus trust. It is an active practice of belief, a solid, unshakeable confidence in God built upon the assurance that he is faithful to his promises.

Take the story of Martha Runyan, for example. Diagnosed with Stargardt disease at age nine, a degenerative macular condition that left her legally blind, Martha refused to let her impairment ruin her life. With the help of special equipment and volunteer readers, she earned two master's degrees at San Diego State University. During this time, she also competed in track events, winning five medals in the Paralympic Games from 1992 to 1999, including the 1,500-meter race at the Pan American Games.

In 2000 and again in 2004, Martha qualified for the U.S. Olympic team, becoming the first legally blind person to compete in the Olympic Games. She placed eighth, the top American women finisher, in the 1,500-meter event in Sydney, Australia. In 2006, she won her second national championship in the 20k event.

Despite her limited peripheral vision, Martha learned to stay in her lane and make the turns on the track. Although she couldn't see how far she had run during the race, she learned to pace herself by listening to the intensity of her competitors' breathing. When asked how she could run toward the finish line she couldn't see, she replied, "I can't see it, but I know it's there." By faith, we move forward even when the destination is not clear.

Faith says that what God has promised will happen. It treats things that are hoped for as a reality. This is described in Hebrews 11:1: "Now faith is the substance of things hoped for, the evidence of things not seen."

Dr. Martin Luther King Jr. expressed this need for trust when he said, "Faith is taking the first step even when you don't see the whole staircase."

How has your faith been tested?

CHAPTER 3: BUILDING HEALTHY RELATIONSHIP

Character of Healthy and Unhealthy Relationship

In an unhealthy relationship, we find ourselves consumed by feelings of clinging and neediness. It's as if our very existence depends on the presence of this person in our lives. We don't match energies with our partners; instead, we often find ourselves giving too much or too little to the relationship, creating an imbalance that breeds resentment and dissatisfaction.

We often suppress or withhold our feelings of anger, fear, and sadness, only to have them erupt in disruptive behaviors such as raging, brooding, or resorting to the silent treatment. These outbursts are often fueled by a desperate attempt to manipulate our partners, acting out of a place of insecurity and emotional turmoil.

In our attempts to control the situation, we fail to align our will with God's will, instead resorting to manipulative tactics to get what we want. We give with ulterior motives, seeking validation and approval from our partners, and becoming crushed when we don't receive it.

As the relationship deteriorates, we begin to neglect our own self-care and withdraw from activities that once brought us joy. We lose sight of who we are as individuals, becoming increasingly reliant on our partner for validation and fulfillment.

Rather than taking responsibility for our own actions, we shift the blame onto our partners, focusing solely on their perceived inadequacies while ignoring our own faults. We expect our partners to make us happy, failing to recognize that true happiness comes from within.

Despite being in the presence of our partner, we feel lonely and isolated, unable to connect on a deeper level due to the toxicity of the relationship. We become obsessed with fixing problems and resolving conflicts, often engaging in circular, no-win arguments that only serve to further damage the relationship.

In summary, an unhealthy relationship is characterized by a lack of balance, emotional manipulation, and a failure to prioritize self-care and individual growth. It's a cycle of dysfunction that perpetuates itself unless we are willing to acknowledge our own shortcomings and take steps to break free from its grip.

Have you ever been involved in an unhealthy relationship?

Healthy Relationship

In a healthy relationship, we find comfort in both the presence and absence of our partner. We feel secure in the connection we share, matching our partner's energy and creating a fluid and enjoyable dynamic.

When feelings of anger or sadness arise, we allow ourselves to feel them fully, recognizing their importance in maintaining a healthy relationship. We communicate these feelings to our partner directly and lovingly, fostering open and honest communication.

We take responsibility for our words and actions, regularly taking inventory and making amends when necessary. We acknowledge our own willfulness and surrender the situation to a higher power, trusting in divine guidance.

In our interactions with our partner, we freely give and receive without expectation, deriving our sense of self-worth from within rather than seeking validation from external sources. We nurture our friendships, engage in hobbies, and prioritize self-care, maintaining a sense of balance and fulfillment in our own lives.

Our sense of self remains intact, and we keep the focus on ourselves rather than placing blame or expectation on our partner. We take responsibility for our own happiness, sharing it with our partner in a mutually supportive and enriching way.

In the presence of our partner, we experience feelings of warmth and intimacy, fostering a deep connection built on trust and mutual respect. We recognize when discussions become destructive and are willing to call for a moratorium to prevent further harm.

Ultimately, we learn to let go of control and trust in a higher power to guide us through challenges and uncertainties. By embracing these principles, we cultivate a relationship grounded in love, understanding, and growth.

A healthy relationship is when you are mature. You must have a relationship with yourself first. Establish boundaries with people. You are able to help people within your own limits. Respect people's time and feelings. Don't give anyone advice if they don't ask for it. They must be emotionally healthy. Healthy people have inner security. They are not always thinking that their worth as a person is on the line. They have the right to be acceptable and valuable. They have respect for the truth. We know that the truth is always based on external values and absolutes. It is the guiding force behind all of your decisions, from big matters, like who you will marry, to little matters.

Always consider the source of the information. If the person is trustworthy or someone who is an alcoholic. Healthy people also know that finding the truth involves collecting all information, allowing all the data to be known so that you can really think. They don't worry about whether your opinion is different from their own. Their security is not threatened by being different. They weigh the information they have collected. They place value on different parts of the information through carefully, although usually unconscious, internal processes that are deeply influenced by well-established moral codes, a value system that informs all decision-making.

Finally, healthy people are authentic; they stand in the middle of the information that they have collected and come to a decision or a position that is a close approximation to the truth with courage and total commitment. They state that position as honestly as they know how and live in accordance with it until they change in light of some new information. Still, they aren't arrogant, assuming that their position and truth are exactly the same. They don't make you feel wrong if you disagree with them. They have a deep humility that seems to emanate from their recognition that they are very fallible; that while they need to come to the best position possible, they also recognize your right to do the same.

How to achieve a healthy Relationship?

Have you ever been involved in a healthy relationship? How can you become healthy if you're not healthy now? But what happens if our parents were anything but healthy? How can you unlearn all the unhealthy ways we picked up from them? Let me make four suggestions about becoming healthy.

Find a source that offers unconditional love, the kind of love you needed when you were a child. Admittedly, good sources for this kind of love are hard to come by. Maybe you can find a close friend or relative. Healthy churches offer unconditional love. The best source of love is the love of God. Wherever you find this kind of love, it is worth everything you have learned to love yourself. It isn't enough that someone else loves you, even if that someone is God. You have to accept the fact that you are lovable when you don't have to fabricate a self in order to please someone else and earn their love. You can just be authentically you.

Find someone who will regularly encourage, inspire, listen, and challenge you. We all need close friends because it is hard, maybe impossible, for us to understand our emotions and know exactly what we're feeling and thinking deep within ourselves. We need someone to help us sort through our thoughts and feelings and help us confront our problems. Cultivate relationships with people who will help you take a stand, be authentic, and feel secure in your position. We all need people who will stay with us, cheer us on, bolster our shaky confidence, and reinforce our courage. An ongoing support system helps us stay on track even when we feel like falling back into unhealthy patterns.

This is what it takes to get ourselves healthy. We need to be reparented in a kind, loving, and thoughtful way by genuinely healthy people. Often these people are friends or family members, but sometimes people need the guidance of well-trained and caring psychotherapists.

What actions have you taken to become healthy? Following are some actions that you can take to achieve a healthy relationship.

Declare your Independence

Spending time alone to get to know the real you in today's constantly connected world has become almost obsolete. There's even a new colloquial term tied to the incessant need to text, tweet, and check our messages: FOMU, or "fear of missing out." But here's a newsflash for your Facebook wall: Solitude is as important as the most fulfilling social connections.

"Western culture tends to view people who spend time alone as sad or antisocial, but there are many benefits to solitude," notes Sherrie Bourg Carter, Psy.D., a psychologist in Fort Lauderdale, Florida, and author of "High Octane Women: How Superachievers Can Avoid

Burnout" (Prometheus Books). Among those benefits, according to research, are freedom, creativity, intimacy, and spirituality.

"Independence and interdependence are both essential," adds Los Angeles psychiatrist Judith Orloff, M.D., author of "Emotional Freedom: Liberate Yourself from Negative Emotions and Transform Your Life" (Harmony Books). It's a balance, but to feel strong and powerful, the relationship with self is the most important relationship you'll ever have. So, declare your independence with these go-solo strategies.

Rise and Shine

Start your day by waking up an hour earlier than the rest of your household, granting yourself a precious hour of solitude. Utilize this quiet time to engage in activities that nourish your soul, whether it's meditation, reading, journaling, or pursuing a hobby that brings you joy.

Sherrie Bourg Carter emphasizes the importance of keeping distractions at bay during this sacred hour. Switch off your phone, resist the urge to check your computer, and leave the television powered down. By eliminating external stimuli, you create a space for deep focus and introspection.

This strategy not only sets a positive tone for your day but also allows you to tackle tasks with renewed clarity and energy. Imagine starting your workday before the hustle and bustle begins, giving you a head start on important projects without interruptions. As Bourg Carter suggests, arriving at work before the usual flurry of activity means you can dive into your tasks before the incessant ringing of phones and flood of emails disrupt your concentration.

Embrace this early morning ritual as a powerful tool for self-care and productivity. By prioritizing quiet time for yourself at the start of each day, you cultivate a sense of balance and inner peace that will carry you through whatever challenges lie ahead.

Set Boundaries

In the quest for emotional well-being, it is particularly crucial to carve out time away from individuals whom Dr. Judith Orloff aptly dubs "emotional vampires." These are people whose interactions tend to leave you feeling drained, upset, or disoriented, as they feed off your energy and often subject you to their own emotional turmoil.

Dr. Orloff notes that engaging with such individuals can evoke a range of negative emotions, including sickness, anger, discomfort, and exhaustion. Their constant drama can even cloud your own sense of identity, as you become entangled in their web of issues and concerns.

While it may be challenging, especially if the emotional vampire is a family member or coworker, Dr. Orloff advises minimizing your exposure to them as much as possible. This might involve setting boundaries, limiting interactions, or finding ways to protect your energy during encounters. However, if the person in question is someone you deem toxic and unnecessary in your life, Dr. Orloff suggests severing ties altogether.

By prioritizing your emotional well-being and distancing yourself from those who drain your energy, you create space for positive relationships and experiences to flourish. Remember, taking care of yourself is not selfish but essential for maintaining your mental and emotional health.

Date Yourself

Sherrie Bourg Carter highlights a common tendency: when in the company of others, we often find ourselves conforming to their desires and preferences. To break free from this pattern, she suggests embracing solo experiences such as dining out, catching a movie, or even embarking on a vacation alone.

Embarking on solo ventures can be eye-opening, providing an opportunity for self-discovery and personal growth. When you're solely responsible for choosing your destination and activities, you gain insight into your own preferences, interests, and desires. Without the influence of others, you're free to follow your instincts and explore new paths.

Venturing out alone allows you to fully immerse yourself in the experience, without the distractions or compromises that often accompany group outings. Whether it's savoring a meal at a new restaurant, indulging in a film that piques your interest, or embarking on an adventure to a destination of your choosing, solo excursions empower you to reconnect with yourself and forge a deeper understanding of who you are.

So, dare to step out of your comfort zone and embrace the freedom of solo exploration. You may be pleasantly surprised by the revelations and discoveries that await you when you take the reins and chart your own course.

What actions have you taken to declare your independence?

CHAPTER 4:
FINANCIAL WELLNESS

Are you feeling the weight of financial strain, struggling to keep up with bills, and receiving daunting notices from creditors? Do thoughts of potential repossession of your home or car loom over you like dark clouds? You're not alone in this predicament. Countless individuals find themselves grappling with financial crises, often triggered by personal or familial illness, sudden job loss, or the all-too-common trap of overspending.

Picture this: you're diligently managing your expenses when an unexpected medical emergency arises, leaving you drowning in unforeseen bills. Or perhaps you've lost your job due to circumstances beyond your control, sending your carefully crafted budget into disarray. Maybe it's the allure of easy credit that led you down a path of accumulating debt, now seemingly insurmountable.

In times like these, it's easy to feel overwhelmed, as if there's no way out. But here's the truth: your financial situation doesn't have to spiral from bad to worse. There are avenues to explore, strategies to employ, and hope to grasp onto. The key lies in understanding your options and taking proactive steps toward financial stability.

Consider this scenario: a close friend confides in you about their mounting debt and their fears of financial ruin. You want to offer support and guidance, but where do you begin? Realistic budgeting, seeking credit counseling from reputable sources, exploring debt consolidation, or even contemplating bankruptcy—these are all potential paths toward relief. But how do you determine which course of action is best suited to your unique circumstances?

The answer isn't straightforward. It hinges on various factors: the extent of your debt, your capacity for discipline and financial management, and your prospects for the future. Each individual's journey to financial wellness is distinct, shaped by personal experiences, challenges, and aspirations.

What steps have you taken to confront your debt head-on?

Let's explore a roadmap to financial well-being, encompassing practical steps and empowering strategies to pave the way toward a brighter financial future.

Develop a Budget

Developing a budget is the cornerstone of financial empowerment, serving as the first step on the path to reclaiming control over your financial well-being. It begins with a candid assessment of your income and expenditures, offering a clear-eyed view of your financial landscape.

Start by meticulously documenting all sources of income, from wages to side hustles, ensuring no revenue stream goes unnoticed. With your income laid bare, turn your attention to expenses. Begin with the fixed costs—the stalwarts of your financial obligations, such as mortgage or rent payments, car expenses, and insurance premiums. These steadfast expenses provide a foundation upon which to build your budget.

But the budgeting process doesn't end there. It's essential to delve deeper, scrutinizing variable expenses like entertainment, recreation, and clothing purchases. Every expenditure, no matter how seemingly inconsequential, deserves a place on your budgetary radar.

Why?

Because understanding your spending patterns empowers you to distinguish between essential needs and discretionary wants, enabling you to allocate your resources judiciously.

The overarching aim? Ensuring your financial solvency by prioritizing the essentials: housing, food, healthcare, insurance, and education. These are the pillars upon which financial stability rests, and your budget should reflect their primacy.

Fortunately, a wealth of resources exists to aid you on your budgeting journey. From books available at your local library to online tutorials and software programs, there's no shortage of tools to assist in crafting and maintaining a budget. These resources not only offer practical guidance but also serve as beacons of support, guiding you through the complexities of money management.

Have you used a budget before?

Contacting Creditors

When facing financial hardship, proactive communication with creditors is paramount. Reach out to them promptly to discuss your circumstances and elucidate why meeting financial obligations has become challenging. Providing a transparent explanation can pave the way for potential solutions and demonstrate your commitment to resolving the situation.

When contacting creditors, be prepared to articulate the factors contributing to your financial strain. Whether it's unexpected medical expenses, a sudden job loss, or a downturn in business, conveying the underlying reasons for your predicament can foster understanding and empathy.

For example, if medical bills have escalated due to an unforeseen illness or injury, share this information with your healthcare provider. Many medical institutions offer financial assistance programs or flexible payment options for patients facing financial hardship. By initiating an open dialogue, you may discover avenues for alleviating the burden of medical debt.

Similarly, if job loss or reduction in income is the culprit, communicate this to your creditors with clarity and honesty. Explain the steps you're taking to secure new employment or explore alternative income sources. Some creditors offer hardship programs or temporary forbearance arrangements to accommodate borrowers experiencing financial setbacks.

It's essential to familiarize yourself with your rights as a debtor, particularly when dealing with debt collectors. The Fair Debt Collection Practices Act (FDCPA) outlines guidelines governing the behavior of debt collectors and safeguards against abusive or deceptive practices.

Under the FDCPA, debt collectors are prohibited from contacting you before 8 a.m. or after 9 p.m., unless you expressly consent to such communications. Moreover, if a debt collector is aware that your employer prohibits personal calls during work hours, they must refrain from contacting you at your place of employment.

Furthermore, debt collectors are prohibited from engaging in harassment, making false statements, or employing unfair tactics to collect a debt. You have the right to request that a debt collector cease further communication with you, and they are obligated to honor such a written request.

Have you contacted your creditors?

Credit Counseling

When navigating the complexities of financial management, maintaining discipline and staying on track can be daunting tasks. If you find yourself struggling to create a viable budget, negotiate repayment plans with creditors, or keep pace with mounting bills, seeking assistance from a credit counseling organization could be a prudent step forward.

Credit counseling organizations, many of which operate as non-profits, specialize in collaborating with individuals to address their financial challenges effectively. However, it's crucial to exercise caution, as the non-profit label doesn't necessarily guarantee free or affordable services, nor does it ensure legitimacy. Some organizations may levy high fees, disguised or pressured as "voluntary contributions," underscoring the importance of due diligence in selecting a reputable provider.

When exploring credit counseling options, prioritize organizations that offer in-person counseling whenever feasible. Many reputable institutions, including universities, military bases, credit unions, housing authorities, and branches of the U.S. Cooperative Extension Service, host counseling programs aimed at fostering financial literacy and empowerment. Additionally, your local consumer protection agency and trusted friends and family can serve as valuable sources of information and referrals.

Reputable credit counseling organizations offer a range of services designed to equip individuals with the tools and knowledge needed to manage their finances effectively. Certified counselors, trained in consumer credit, money management, debt management, and budgeting, engage clients in comprehensive discussions to assess their financial landscape thoroughly.

During an initial counseling session, which typically lasts about an hour, counselors delve into your entire financial situation, from income and expenses to debt obligations and savings goals. Through this collaborative process, counselors work with you to develop a personalized action plan tailored to address your specific financial challenges.

Furthermore, credit counseling organizations extend ongoing support beyond the initial session, offering follow-up consultations and educational workshops to reinforce financial literacy and empower informed decision-making.

So, if you're grappling with financial uncertainty and seeking guidance on managing your money and debt, consider reaching out to a reputable credit counseling organization. With their expertise and support, you can embark on a journey toward financial stability and peace of mind.

Have you thought about credit counseling?

Auto and Home Loans

When it comes to managing debt, understanding the distinction between secured and unsecured debts is crucial. Secured debts, such as auto loans and mortgages, are typically tied to specific assets—your car for an auto loan or your house for a mortgage. In the event of default, lenders have the legal right to repossess the asset, leading to potential consequences like foreclosure on your home or repossession of your vehicle.

On the other hand, unsecured debts are not backed by any collateral and include obligations like credit card debt, medical bills, signature loans, and service-related debts. While creditors cannot seize specific assets for unsecured debts, they may pursue other avenues, such as wage garnishment or legal action, to recover what is owed.

When it comes to auto loans, it's essential to be aware of your creditor's rights in the event of default. Most automobile financing agreements grant creditors the authority to repossess your car without prior notice if you fall behind on payments. Should repossession occur, you may be liable for the outstanding balance on the loan, along with additional expenses such as towing and storage fees. In some cases, selling the car yourself before defaulting on the loan could mitigate these costs and prevent negative entries on your credit report.

Similarly, if you find yourself struggling to keep up with mortgage payments, swift action is imperative to avoid foreclosure. Contact your lender at the earliest sign of financial distress to explore potential solutions. Many lenders are willing to collaborate with borrowers facing temporary setbacks, offering options such as payment suspension or modification of loan terms. However, it's essential to assess the long-term implications of any proposed changes, including potential fees and adjustments to the repayment period.

If negotiations with your lender prove unsuccessful, seeking assistance from a housing counseling agency can provide invaluable support. These agencies specialize in assisting homeowners facing mortgage challenges, offering guidance on navigating the complex landscape of foreclosure prevention and loan modification. To locate a reputable housing counseling agency in your area, reach out to local offices of the Department of Housing and Urban Development or housing authorities for assistance.

By understanding your rights and exploring available resources, you can take proactive steps to mitigate the impact of auto and home loan debt, safeguarding your financial stability in the process.

Have you taken an auto or home loan?

Debt Consolidation

Debt consolidation can offer a potential solution for individuals burdened by high-interest credit card debt, providing an opportunity to streamline payments and potentially reduce overall costs. One common method of consolidation involves leveraging the equity in your home through a second mortgage or a home equity line of credit (HELOC). However, it's crucial to approach these options with caution, as they entail using your home as collateral.

By consolidating debt with a second mortgage or HELOC, you essentially combine multiple high-interest debts into a single, more manageable payment. This can simplify your financial obligations and potentially lower your overall interest rate, leading to savings over time. However, it's essential to weigh the benefits against the risks, particularly the potential loss of your home if you default on payments.

Furthermore, it's important to consider the associated costs of consolidation loans. In addition to interest charges, you may be required to pay points, with each point representing one percent of the loan amount. These upfront costs can impact the overall affordability of the loan and should be factored into your decision-making process.

Despite the potential drawbacks, consolidation loans secured by your home may offer certain tax advantages not available with other forms of credit. Interest payments on mortgage-related debt may be tax-deductible in some circumstances, providing a potential financial benefit for homeowners.

Before pursuing debt consolidation, it's essential to carefully assess your financial situation and consider alternative options. Evaluate whether consolidation aligns with your long-term financial goals and whether you have the means to meet the associated payment obligations consistently. Additionally, explore alternative methods of debt management, such as budgeting, negotiating with creditors, or seeking assistance from non-profit credit counseling agencies.

Ultimately, debt consolidation can be a valuable tool for some individuals seeking to regain control of their finances. However, it's not without risks, and careful consideration of the potential benefits and drawbacks is essential to making an informed decision. By weighing your options carefully and seeking professional guidance if needed, you can take steps toward a more stable financial future.

Do you find debt consolidation helpful or hurtful?

Bankruptcy

Filing for personal bankruptcy is often viewed as a last resort for managing overwhelming debt, primarily due to its far-reaching consequences. A bankruptcy filing can have a profound and long-lasting impact on your financial life, including a significant hit to your credit score that can linger for up to 10 years. This may hinder your ability to obtain credit, secure a mortgage, acquire life insurance, or even land certain job opportunities.

However, despite its drawbacks, bankruptcy is a legal process designed to offer relief to individuals who find themselves unable to meet their financial obligations. By following the bankruptcy rules, individuals may receive a discharge—a court order absolving them from repaying certain debts. It's important to note that the consequences of bankruptcy are substantial and require careful consideration of both the benefits and drawbacks.

In October 2005, Congress implemented significant changes to the bankruptcy laws, affecting both consumers and creditors. These changes aimed to provide consumers with more incentives to seek relief under Chapter 13 bankruptcy. Under Chapter 13, individuals with a steady income have the opportunity to retain valuable assets, such as a mortgaged home or car, by adhering to a court-approved repayment plan over a three to five-year period.

Conversely, Chapter 7 bankruptcy, often referred to as straight bankruptcy, involves the liquidation of non-exempt assets to repay creditors. While some assets may be exempt from liquidation, such as work-related tools or basic household furnishings, others may be sold by a court-appointed trustee to satisfy outstanding debts.

After receiving a discharge through Chapter 7 bankruptcy, individuals must wait eight years before they can file for bankruptcy under the same chapter again. In contrast, the waiting period for Chapter 13 bankruptcy is typically shorter, allowing individuals to file again after as little as two years.

It's important to understand that while bankruptcy may eliminate certain unsecured debts and halt debt collection activities, it does not erase obligations such as child support, alimony, taxes, fines, or some student loans. Additionally, bankruptcy may not allow individuals to retain property secured by unpaid mortgages or liens unless they have a viable plan to catch up on payments.

Before filing for bankruptcy, individuals must fulfill certain requirements, including receiving credit counseling from a government-approved organization within six months of filing. Additionally, those considering Chapter 7 bankruptcy must pass a means test to ensure their income does not exceed certain thresholds, which vary by state.

Navigating the complexities of bankruptcy requires careful consideration and professional guidance. It's essential to weigh the potential benefits and consequences thoroughly before proceeding with a bankruptcy filing.

Have you thought about bankruptcy?

Covering the terrain of financial wellness requires diligence, resilience, and informed decision-making. Throughout this chapter, we've explored various strategies and avenues for managing debt, from developing a realistic budget to considering options such as credit counseling, debt consolidation, and bankruptcy.

It's important to recognize that each individual's financial journey is unique, shaped by personal circumstances, challenges, and aspirations. While there is no one-size-fits-all solution to achieving financial stability, arming yourself with knowledge and resources can empower you to make sound financial decisions and chart a path toward a brighter future.

Whether you're grappling with mounting debt, facing unexpected financial setbacks, or striving to build a stronger financial foundation, remember that you are not alone. Seeking assistance from reputable sources, such as credit counseling agencies, financial advisors, or legal professionals, can provide invaluable support and guidance along the way.

Ultimately, the road to financial wellness is a journey—one that requires patience, perseverance, and a commitment to taking proactive steps toward a more secure financial future. By implementing the principles and strategies outlined in this chapter, you can overcome financial challenges, regain control of your finances, and pave the way for a life of financial freedom and security.

CHAPTER 5:
WHAT DOES A BOUNDARY LOOK LIKE?

Invisible Property Lines and Responsibility

In the tangible realm, property boundaries are clearly demarcated by physical structures like fences, signs, walls, or even the occasional moat with alligators. These visible markers communicate a simple message: "THIS IS WHERE MY PROPERTY BEGINS." Legally, property owners bear responsibility for what occurs within their boundaries, while non-owners are absolved of such obligations. These physical boundaries serve as tangible indicators of property ownership, often delineated in official property deeds accessible at the county courthouse. Understanding these boundaries is crucial for knowing whom to contact regarding property-related matters.

In the spiritual realm, boundaries are equally significant but less conspicuous. Here, boundaries define the contours of your soul, safeguarding and preserving its integrity. Though intangible, these boundaries play a vital role in maintaining spiritual well-being.

Just as physical boundaries shield property, spiritual boundaries serve to protect the essence of who you are. They delineate what is acceptable and what is not, guiding your interactions and safeguarding your emotional and mental health. Establishing and upholding these boundaries is essential for fostering self-respect, maintaining healthy relationships, and nurturing personal growth.

While physical boundaries may be readily visible, spiritual boundaries require introspection and self-awareness to discern. Yet, just as property owners rely on tangible markers to assert ownership, individuals must cultivate inner clarity and assertiveness to uphold their spiritual boundaries.

In essence, understanding and respecting both physical and spiritual boundaries is fundamental to navigating life with integrity and purpose. By acknowledging and honoring these invisible lines of responsibility, we can cultivate a deeper sense of self-awareness, foster healthier relationships, and safeguard our well-being in both the material and immaterial realms.

Me and Not Me: Understanding Boundaries

Boundaries define us. They distinguish what is "me" from what is "not me." A boundary serves as a marker, indicating where I end and someone else begins, granting me a sense of ownership and responsibility. Knowing what I am accountable for in my life opens up a multitude of possibilities. However, if I fail to take ownership of my life, my choices, and my actions, my options become severely limited. Imagine being entrusted with the task of guarding a property diligently, yet not being informed of its boundaries or provided with the means to protect it. Such a scenario would not only be confusing but potentially dangerous.

This analogy mirrors our emotional and spiritual reality. God has crafted a world in which we inhabit our own souls, each responsible for the state of our being. As Proverbs 14:10 aptly states, "The heart knows its own bitterness, and no one shares its joy." We must contend with the contents of our souls, and boundaries play a crucial role in defining and safeguarding our inner world. Without clear parameters, or when taught erroneous boundaries, we are destined to experience profound anguish.

Thankfully, the Bible offers clear guidance on our spiritual boundaries and how to protect them. However, familial or societal influences can often obscure our understanding of these fundamental principles.

In addition to delineating our responsibilities, boundaries also help us discern what is not within our purview. We are not, for instance, accountable for the actions or emotions of others. Nowhere in Scripture are we instructed to exercise "other-control," yet we expend significant time and energy attempting to do so.

Understanding and respecting boundaries is paramount for cultivating self-awareness, nurturing healthy relationships, and preserving emotional well-being. By embracing our responsibility for ourselves and recognizing the limitations of our influence, we can navigate life with clarity, confidence, and integrity.

To and For: Understanding Responsibility

We bear a dual responsibility: to others and for ourselves. Galatians 6:2 instructs us to "carry each other's burdens," emphasizing our duty to assist and support one another, thereby fulfilling the law of Christ. This verse underscores our obligation to extend a helping hand to those overwhelmed by burdens too weighty to bear alone. In embodying sacrificial love, we mirror the selfless example set by Christ, who bore our burdens and saved us when we were incapable of doing so ourselves. This exemplifies being responsible "to" others.

Conversely, verse 5 of the same chapter asserts that "each one should carry their own load," highlighting the individual responsibilities that each person must shoulder. These personal responsibilities constitute our unique "load," requiring daily attention and effort to manage effectively. While others can offer support and guidance, certain tasks are inherently ours to fulfill.

Examining the Greek words for "burden" and "load" provides deeper insight into these concepts. The Greek term for "burden" denotes excessive weights or crushing burdens that can overwhelm us, akin to boulders that threaten to crush our spirits. In times of crisis or tragedy, these burdens are too heavy to bear alone, necessitating assistance and communal support.

In contrast, the Greek word for "load" refers to the daily responsibilities and toils of life, akin to cargo or knapsacks that are manageable to carry. These are the routine tasks, feelings, attitudes, and behaviors that form part of our daily existence and require our individual attention and effort.

Problems arise when individuals misconstrue their burdens as daily loads or refuse assistance when overwhelmed by burdens. Such misconceptions lead to either enduring suffering or shirking responsibility.

To avoid perpetual pain or irresponsibility, it is imperative to delineate our boundaries of responsibility—where "me" ends and another begins. While we will delve deeper into defining our responsibilities later in this chapter, it is essential to first understand the nature of boundaries and their significance in navigating life with clarity and integrity.

Good In, Bad Out: Boundaries For Protection

Boundaries serve as protective fences around our hearts and lives, allowing us to nurture and safeguard what is valuable within. They are essential for maintaining our well-being, as they enable us to discern what should be kept inside and what should be kept out. In the words of Matthew 7:6, boundaries protect our treasures from being stolen, ensuring that pearls remain within while keeping the influence of pigs at bay.

At times, however, our internal landscape may be marred by pain or sin that needs to be addressed. In such instances, we must be willing to open the gates of our boundaries and confess our struggles to God and others, allowing healing to take place (1 John 1:9; James 5:16; Mark 7:21-23).

Conversely, when goodness and truth are present outside our boundaries, we must be open to receiving them. Jesus invites us to "receive" him and his truth (Revelation 3:20; John 1:12), while Paul encourages us to open our hearts to others (2 Corinthians 6:11-13). Closing ourselves off from the positive influences of others can lead to a state of deprivation and isolation.

It's important to note that boundaries are not meant to be impenetrable walls. Rather, they should be permeable enough to allow healthy interactions while still providing protection from harm. However, when individuals have experienced abuse or trauma, they may inadvertently reverse the function of their boundaries, keeping the bad in and shutting out the good.

Take Mary, for example, who endured abuse during her upbringing. Lacking healthy boundaries, she internalized her pain and closed herself off from seeking help or support. In order to heal, Mary needed boundaries that could effectively keep out harmful influences while allowing her to release the pain within and receive the support she desperately needed.

In essence, maintaining healthy boundaries involves finding the balance between protection and openness, ensuring that we can safeguard our well-being while remaining receptive to the positive influences of the world around us.

God and Boundaries: Embracing Divine Example

The concept of boundaries finds its origins in the very nature of God Himself. God defines Himself as a distinct and separate being, assuming responsibility for His own character and actions. He reveals His thoughts, feelings, plans, and preferences, delineating who He is and what He stands for. Moreover, God establishes Himself as separate from His creation and from us, clearly distinguishing His identity from that of others. For instance, He proclaims Himself as love while rejecting darkness (1 John 4:16; 1:6).

Within the Trinity, God exemplifies boundaries in perfect harmony. Though the Father, Son, and Holy Spirit are unified as one, each person maintains distinct personhood and responsibilities while sharing a profound connection and love for one another (John 17:24).

God exercises discernment in what He allows within His realm, confronting sin and administering consequences for behavior. He maintains the sanctity of His domain, inviting those who embrace His love while barring the intrusion of evil. The "gates" of His boundaries open and close appropriately, ensuring the flow of love and protection.

In extending His likeness to humanity (Genesis 1:26), God entrusts us with personal responsibility within defined limits. He charges us to rule and steward the earth, urging us to be faithful caretakers of the life He has bestowed upon us. To fulfill this mandate, we are called to emulate God's example by cultivating boundaries that reflect His wisdom and grace.

Examples of Boundaries

Boundaries encompass anything that distinguishes you from others, signaling where you begin and end. Here are some illustrative examples of boundaries:

Skin

Your physical skin is perhaps the most fundamental boundary that defines you. It serves as the barrier between your internal and external environment, safeguarding your blood, bones, and vital organs. Metaphorically, people often refer to having their "personal boundaries violated," akin to someone "getting under their skin." From infancy, we learn that our physical selves are separate from those around us, as demonstrated when a baby gradually recognizes their individuality distinct from their caregivers. The skin boundary functions to keep the good in and the bad out, shielding us from germs and infection while allowing essential nutrients to enter and waste products to exit. However, victims of physical or sexual abuse may struggle to establish healthy boundaries, having learned early in life that their personal space was not respected.

Words

In the physical realm, boundaries are often demarcated by fences or structures. Conversely, in the spiritual realm, boundaries are intangible but can be established through language. The word "no" is a fundamental boundary-setting tool, asserting your autonomy and signaling that you are in control of yourself. Throughout the Bible, the importance of clarity in stating "no" and "yes" is emphasized (Matthew 5:37; James 5:12). Saying "no" is crucial for confronting inappropriate behavior and setting limits on abuse, as encouraged by various passages of scripture (Matthew 18:15-20).

People with poor boundaries often struggle to assert themselves and say "no," fearing conflict or jeopardizing relationships. Yet, failing to set boundaries leads to resentment and a loss of self-control. Your words also serve to communicate your feelings, intentions, and dislikes, defining your personal space for others. By expressing your preferences and boundaries, you provide clarity and establish the "edges" that help others understand and respect your individuality. For example, stating, "I don't like it when you yell at me!" communicates your boundaries and sets expectations for how you wish to be treated in relationships.

Truth

Understanding the truth about God and His domain sets boundaries for us and reveals His divine limits. Recognizing the unchangeable reality of God's truth allows us to define ourselves in relation to Him. For instance, when God declares that we will reap what we sow (Galatians 6:7), we must either align ourselves with this reality or face the consequences of disregarding it. Being in tune with God's truth means living in harmony with reality, leading to a more fulfilling life (Psalm 119:2,45).

In contrast, Satan seeks to distort reality, as seen in the Garden of Eden when he tempted Eve to question God's boundaries and truth, resulting in dire consequences. Hence, embracing the truth offers a sanctuary of safety, whether it involves understanding God's truth, acknowledging the truth about ourselves, or living within our personal boundaries. Many individuals lead chaotic lives because they resist accepting and expressing the truth of who they are. Honesty about our identity grants us the biblical virtue of integrity, fostering a sense of oneness within ourselves and with God's divine order.

Geographical Distance

Proverbs 22:3 advises that "the prudent man sees evil and hides himself." At times, physically distancing yourself from a situation becomes essential to uphold boundaries. This separation allows for physical, emotional, and spiritual rejuvenation, similar to how Jesus often retreated to solitary places after periods of intense ministry.

Moreover, removing yourself from danger is a proactive measure to establish boundaries and protect yourself from harm. The Bible encourages separation from individuals who persistently inflict harm, emphasizing the importance of creating a safe environment (Matthew 18:17-18; 1 Corinthians 5:11-13). By withdrawing from toxic relationships, you not only safeguard your well-being but also signal to the other party the seriousness of your boundaries. This separation may prompt introspection and behavioral change in the individual left behind.

In cases of abuse, creating distance may be the only effective means to demonstrate the reality of your boundaries and encourage accountability. The biblical principle of limiting togetherness for the purpose of restraining evil underscores the necessity of prioritizing personal safety and well-being. By implementing geographical distance, individuals assert their right to boundaries and establish healthier relational dynamics.

Time

Allocating time away from certain individuals or projects can serve as a strategic approach to reestablishing control over areas of life where boundaries need reinforcement. This intentional break allows individuals to regain ownership of aspects that may have become overwhelming or blurred.

For adult children who have yet to achieve spiritual and emotional independence from their parents, taking time apart becomes crucial. Often, these individuals have spent their entire lives enmeshed in familial dynamics, hesitant to deviate from familiar patterns (Ecclesiastes 3:5-6). By temporarily distancing themselves, they create space to redefine boundaries, shedding outdated modes of interaction and cultivating healthier relational dynamics. While this separation may initially feel disorienting or unsettling, it ultimately fosters personal growth and enhances the quality of their relationship with their parents.

Emotional Distance

Emotional distance serves as a temporary boundary, providing your heart with the necessary space to heal and safeguard itself. However, it is not intended to be a permanent lifestyle choice. Individuals who have endured abusive relationships often require a safe environment to begin emotionally thawing out. In cases of abusive marriages, the victimized spouse may need to maintain emotional distance until the abusive partner acknowledges their issues and demonstrates genuine efforts towards change and trustworthiness.

Continuously subjecting oneself to hurt and disappointment is neither advisable nor sustainable. If you have experienced abuse in a relationship, it is imperative to prioritize your safety and well-being. Before considering reconciliation, it is essential to wait until it is safe to do so and until tangible patterns of positive change have been established. Rushing back into a relationship without witnessing genuine transformation is unwise, as forgiveness should not come at the expense of self-preservation (Luke 3:8). While forgiveness is crucial, it must be accompanied by prudent guarding of one's heart until sustained change is evident.

Other People

Establishing boundaries often requires support from others, especially for individuals who have endured addiction, control, or abuse from another person. After years of tolerating unhealthy dynamics, many individuals find the strength to create boundaries only through the guidance and encouragement of a supportive community or group. This external support system empowers them to assert themselves and say no to abuse and manipulation for the first time.

There are two primary reasons why seeking assistance from others is essential in boundary setting. Firstly, human beings have an inherent need for relationships, and the fear of abandonment often compels individuals to endure mistreatment rather than risk being alone. However, by embracing support from others, individuals realize that love and companionship are not solely dependent on the abusive individual. This newfound sense of community provides them with the courage and resilience needed to establish healthy boundaries and break free from harmful patterns.

Secondly, seeking external support is crucial for acquiring new perspectives and teachings. Many individuals have been influenced by erroneous beliefs propagated by their church or family, viewing boundaries as ungodly, selfish, or mean. Such ingrained misconceptions can lead to feelings of guilt and resistance to change. Therefore, a robust support network, rooted in biblical principles, becomes indispensable in challenging these outdated ideologies and fostering personal growth and empowerment.

In the subsequent discussion in Part 2, we will delve deeper into the process of building boundaries within various primary relationships. However, it is vital to emphasize that boundary setting does not occur in isolation; it necessitates the presence of a supportive community or network to provide guidance, encouragement, and accountability along the journey.

Consequences

Just as "No Trespassing" signs carry the threat of prosecution for crossing property boundaries, the Bible consistently emphasizes the principle of cause and effect, detailing the consequences of various actions. In our personal lives, it becomes imperative to reinforce our boundaries with consequences, ensuring that our limits are respected and upheld.

Consider how many marriages might have been salvaged if one spouse had followed through on their ultimatum: "If you don't seek treatment for your drinking, coming home late, or abusive behavior, I will leave until you do." Similarly, imagine the potential for positive change in the lives of young adults if parents had enforced consequences for irresponsible behavior, such as withholding financial support until they secured stable employment or prohibiting certain behaviors within the household.

In 2 Thessalonians 3:10, the apostle Paul underscores the importance of accountability and responsibility by stating that those who refuse to work should not be given food. This passage highlights the biblical principle that God does not enable irresponsible behavior, and that experiencing hunger can serve as a natural consequence of laziness (Proverbs 16:26).

Implementing consequences adds strength to our boundaries, serving as a deterrent to boundary violations and signaling the seriousness of our self-respect and values. By establishing and enforcing consequences, we communicate our commitment to maintaining healthy boundaries and safeguarding our well-being.

What's Within My Boundaries?

The parable of the Good Samaritan offers profound insights into the complexities of boundaries and their impact on our behavior. This timeless story, often celebrated for its message of compassion, also prompts us to consider the nuances of setting and respecting personal boundaries.

Picture this familiar scene: a man, beaten and left for dead by the side of the road, receives aid from an unlikely Samaritan after being ignored by religious figures. Now, let's pause the narrative and imagine a different scenario—one in which the Samaritan lacks clear boundaries.

As the Samaritan tends to the wounded man, he abruptly announces his departure to attend to business in Jericho, leaving the injured individual bewildered and abandoned.

"What? You're leaving?" the injured man exclaims, his voice tinged with disbelief.

"Yes, I am. I have some business in Jericho I have to attend to," the Samaritan replies matter-of-factly.

"Don't you think you're being selfish? I'm in pretty bad shape here. I'm going to need someone to talk to. How is Jesus going to use you as an example? You're not even acting like a Christian, abandoning me like this in my time of need! Whatever happened to 'Deny yourself'?" the wounded man protests, his tone pleading.

"Why, I guess you're right," the Samaritan concedes, his expression troubled. "That would be uncaring of me to leave you here alone. I should do more. I will postpone my trip for a few days."

So he stays with the man for three days, talking to him and making sure that he is happy and content. On the afternoon of the third day, there's a knock at the door and a messenger comes in.

He hands the Samaritan a message from his business contacts in Jericho: "Waited as long as could. Have decided to sell camels to another party. Our next herd will be here in six months."

"How could you do this to me?" the Samaritan screams at the recovering man, waving the message in the air. "Look what you've done now! You caused me to lose those camels that I needed for my business. Now I can't deliver my goods. This may put me out of business! How could you do this to me?"

This alternate narrative serves as a poignant reminder of the challenges inherent in navigating boundaries. While the Samaritan's initial impulse to help is commendable, his failure to establish clear limits leads to resentment and frustration for both parties involved.

This story may resonate with many of us, as we grapple with the delicate balance of compassion and self-preservation in our interactions with others. We may find ourselves compelled to give generously, only to feel manipulated or taken advantage of in return. Conversely, when we demand more than others can give, we risk damaging relationships and fostering resentment.

To avoid these pitfalls, we must cultivate a deeper understanding of our own boundaries and responsibilities. By recognizing and respecting our limits, we can foster healthier, more authentic connections built on mutual respect and genuine care. In doing so, we empower ourselves and others to navigate relationships with integrity and compassion, ensuring that everyone's needs are honored and respected.

Feelings

Feelings often receive a contentious reception within Christian circles. They're sometimes dismissed as inconsequential or even sinful. Yet, countless examples demonstrate their profound influence on our actions and attitudes. How often have we witnessed individuals commit hurtful acts due to wounded feelings? Or seen others spiral into depression after years of suppressing their emotions, until despair becomes overwhelming?

However, feelings shouldn't be disregarded or given unchecked authority. Scripture encourages us to acknowledge and understand our emotions. They can serve as powerful motivators for good deeds. Consider the Good Samaritan, whose compassion moved him to assist the injured Israelite (Luke 10:33). Similarly, the father in the parable of the prodigal son was filled with compassion for his wayward child and embraced him warmly (Luke 15:20). Jesus himself frequently demonstrated compassion towards those he ministered to (Matthew 9:36; 15:32).

Feelings originate from the heart and offer insights into the state of our relationships. They signal whether things are harmonious or if issues need addressing. Feeling close and affectionate often indicates a healthy connection, while anger may signify unresolved problems. Yet, crucially, our feelings are our own responsibility. We must take ownership of them and recognize them as indicators of issues that require attention and resolution. Only then can we begin to find solutions to the challenges they reveal.

Attitudes and Beliefs

Attitudes pertain to your orientation toward others, God, life, work, and relationships. Beliefs encompass anything you accept as true. Often, we fail to recognize attitudes or beliefs as sources of discomfort in our lives. Like our first parents, Adam and Eve, we tend to attribute blame to others. However, it's essential to take ownership of our attitudes and convictions because they fall within our property line. We are the ones who feel their effects, and we are the only ones who can change them.

The challenging aspect of attitudes is that we acquire them at a very early age. They significantly influence who we are and how we navigate the world. Those who have never questioned their attitudes and beliefs may become ensnared in the dynamic Jesus referred to when he spoke of people adhering to "the traditions of men" rather than the commands of God (Mark 7:8; Matthew 15:3).

Individuals with boundary issues often harbor distorted attitudes about responsibility. They perceive holding others accountable for their feelings, choices, and behaviors as unkind. However, Proverbs repeatedly emphasizes that setting limits and embracing responsibility can save lives (Proverbs 13:18, 24).

Behaviors

Behaviors have consequences, as Paul articulates, "A man reaps what he sows" (Galatians 6:7-8). If we diligently study, we will reap good grades. If we fulfill our work responsibilities, we will receive a paycheck. If we prioritize exercise, we will enjoy better health. Acting lovingly towards others fosters closer relationships. Conversely, engaging in idleness, irresponsibility, or uncontrolled behavior leads to negative outcomes such as poverty, failure, and the repercussions of reckless living. These are the natural consequences of our actions.

The issue arises when individuals intervene in the law of sowing and reaping in another's life. Drinking or abusive behavior should entail consequences for the individual engaging in such actions. "Stern discipline awaits him who leaves the path" (Proverbs 15:10). Rescuing people from the natural consequences of their behavior renders them powerless.

This scenario commonly unfolds between parents and children. Instead of allowing their children to face the natural outcomes of their actions, parents often resort to yelling and nagging. Parenting with a balance of love and boundaries, warmth and consequences, fosters the development of confident children who feel empowered to manage their lives.

Choices

Taking responsibility for our choices is essential. This cultivates the fruit of "self-control" (Galatians 5:23). A prevalent boundary issue involves disowning our choices and attributing responsibility to others. Consider how often we use phrases like "I had to" or "She (he) made me" to deflect accountability for our actions. Such phrases reveal our fundamental misconception that we are not active agents in our dealings and shift blame to external factors.

We must recognize that we are in control of our choices, irrespective of our emotions. This prevents us from making decisions reluctantly or under compulsion, as noted in 2 Corinthians 9:7. Paul refused to accept gifts given out of obligation, emphasizing the importance of spontaneous giving (Philemon 1:14). Similarly, Joshua urged the people to make a deliberate choice regarding whom they would serve (Joshua 24:15).

Jesus reiterated this principle when addressing the disgruntled worker who felt unfairly compensated for his labor (Matthew 20:13). The worker had voluntarily agreed to a wage but became resentful when others received the same pay for fewer hours worked. Likewise, the prodigal son's brother chose to remain at home and serve, yet harbored resentment. He was reminded that his decision was his own.

Throughout Scripture, individuals are reminded of their choices and urged to take responsibility for them. As Paul emphasizes, choosing to live by the Spirit leads to life, whereas following the sinful nature leads to death (Romans 8:13). Making decisions based on others' approval or guilt fosters resentment, a byproduct of our sinful nature. We often feel compelled to act in certain ways due to external pressure or expectations, believing it to be an expression of love.

Setting boundaries inevitably entails taking responsibility for our choices. We must live with their consequences and recognize that we may be hindering ourselves from making choices that would bring us contentment.

Values

What we value is what we love and assign importance to. Often, we fail to take responsibility for our values, becoming ensnared in the pursuit of human approval rather than God's (John 12:43). This misplaced value system leads us astray, as we mistakenly believe that power, wealth, and pleasure will satisfy our deepest longings, which are truly for love.

Taking responsibility for our out-of-control behavior, stemming from misplaced or transient values, begins with acknowledging that our hearts prioritize things that ultimately fail to satisfy. By confessing our inclination towards fleeting values, we open ourselves to God's transformative work in creating a new heart within us. Boundaries serve not to deny but to own our harmful values, allowing God to initiate change within us.

Limits

Two fundamental aspects of limits emerge in the context of establishing healthier boundaries. Firstly, there's setting limits on others, a concept commonly associated with boundary discussions. However, the notion of imposing limits on others is misleading; we cannot dictate or compel their behavior. Instead, we can only control our own exposure to individuals exhibiting inappropriate conduct. Much like God, who establishes standards but grants individuals agency, we can delineate boundaries by separating ourselves from those who engage in misconduct. This separation serves to protect love by taking a stand against behaviors that undermine it.

The other crucial aspect of limits concerns setting internal boundaries. It's imperative to establish internal spaces within ourselves where feelings, impulses, or desires can exist without immediate action. This entails the ability to exercise self-restraint, saying no to both destructive urges and well-intentioned desires that may not be prudent at a given moment. Internal structure forms a vital component of boundaries and identity, encompassing ownership, responsibility, and self-control.

Talents

Contrast these two responses:

"Well done, good and faithful servant! You have been faithful with a few things; I will put you in charge of many things. Come and share your master's happiness!"

"You wicked, lazy servant! So you knew that I harvest where I have not sown and gather where I have not scattered seed? Then you should have put my money on deposit with the bankers, so that when I returned I would have received it back with interest. Take the talent from him and give it to the one who has the ten talents." (Matthew 25:23, 26-28)

No other passage better illustrates God-ordained responsibility for the ownership and use of talents. Although the example is of money, it also applies to internal talents and gifts. Our talents are clearly within our boundaries and are our responsibility. Yet, taking ownership of them is often frightening and always risky.

The parable of the talents says that we are accountable, not to mention much happier, when we are exercising our gifts and being productive. It takes work, practice, learning, prayer, resources, and grace to overcome the fear of failure that the "wicked and lazy" servant gave in to. He was not chastised for being afraid when trying something new and difficult. He was chastised for not confronting his fear and trying the best he could. Not confronting our fear denies the grace of God and insults both his giving of the gift and his grace to sustain us as we are learning.

Thoughts

Our minds and thoughts are important reflections of the image of God. No other creature on earth has our thinking ability. We are the only creatures who are called to love God with all our mind (Mark 12:30). And Paul wrote that he was taking "captive every thought to make it obedient to Christ" (2 Cor. 10:5). Establishing boundaries in thinking involves three things:

1. We must know our own thoughts. Many people have not taken ownership of their own thinking processes. They mechanically think the thoughts of others without ever examining them. They swallow others' opinions and reasonings without questioning and "thinking about their thinking". Certainly, we should listen to the thoughts of others and weigh them; but we should never "give our minds" over to anyone.

2. We must grow in knowledge and expand our minds. One area in which we need to grow is in the knowledge of God and his Word. David said of knowing God's Word, "My soul

is consumed with longing for your laws at all times. Your statutes are my delight; they are my counselors" (Psalm 119:20, 24). We also learn much about God by studying his creation and his work. In learning about his world, we obey the commandment to "rule and subdue" the earth and all that is within it. We must learn about the world that he has given us to become wise stewards. Whether we are dealing with brain injuries, balancing our checkbooks, or raising children, we are to use our brains to lead better lives and glorify God.

3. We must clarify distorted thinking. We all have a tendency to not see things clearly, to think and perceive in distorted ways. Probably the easiest distortions to notice are in personal relationships. We rarely see people as they really are; our perceptions are distorted by past relationships and our own preconceptions of who we think they are, even the people we know best. We do not see clearly because of the "logs" in our eyes (Matthew 7:3-5).

Taking ownership of our thinking in relationships requires actively checking where we may be wrong. As we assimilate new information, our thinking adapts and grows closer to reality.

Also, we need to ensure that we are communicating our thoughts to others. Many people think that others should be able to read their minds and know what they want. This leads to frustration. Even Paul says, "For who among men knows the thoughts of a man except the man's own spirit within him?" (1 Corinthians 2:11). What a great statement about boundaries! We have our own thoughts, and if we want others to know them, we must tell them.

Desires

Our desires reside within the boundaries of our being. Each of us harbors different longings, dreams, aspirations, and cravings. We all seek satisfaction, but do we truly understand the nature of our desires?

Part of the challenge stems from the lack of well-defined boundaries within our personalities. Without clarity on who the authentic "me" is and what we genuinely desire, many of our wants masquerade as genuine needs. These desires often emerge from unacknowledged yearnings. For instance, individuals struggling with sex addiction may pursue sexual encounters, but at the core, what they truly crave is love and affection.

James addresses this issue of pursuing desires with impure motives: "You desire but do not have, so you kill. You covet but you cannot get what you want, so you quarrel and fight. You do not have because you do not ask God. When you ask, you do not receive, because you ask with wrong motives, that you may spend what you get on your pleasures" (James 4:2-3). Often, we fail to seek our desires from God, and when we do, they are entangled with unnecessary wants. However, God is genuinely interested in our desires; after all, He created them. Consider the following: "You have granted him his heart's desire and have not withheld the request of his lips. You welcomed him with rich blessings and placed a crown of pure gold on his head" (Psalm 21:2-3). "Delight yourself in the Lord, and he will give you the desires of your heart" (Psalm 37:4). "He fulfills the desires of those who fear him" (Psalm 145:19).

God delights in giving gifts to His children, but as a wise parent, He ensures His gifts are suitable for us. To discern what to ask for, we must be in tune with our true selves and examine our motives. If our desires stem from pride or ego, it's unlikely that God will grant them. However, if they align with His will, He is eager to fulfill them.

Moreover, Scripture instructs us to actively pursue our desires (Philippians 2:12-13; Ecclesiastes 11:9; Matthew 7:7-11). We must take ownership of our desires and diligently pursue them to find fulfillment in life. As Proverbs 13:19 states, "A desire fulfilled is sweet to the soul," but it requires effort and commitment.

Love

Our capacity to give and receive love is perhaps our most profound gift. The heart, crafted in the image of God, serves as the core of our being, facilitating our ability to both embrace love and extend it outward. Yet, for many, the journey of loving and being loved is hindered by past hurts and present fears, resulting in closed hearts and a sense of emptiness. Scripture aptly delineates the dual role of the heart: to receive love and grace inwardly, and to radiate love outwardly.

Consider the biblical exhortations on love: "Love the Lord your God with all your heart and with all your soul and with all your mind... Love your neighbor as yourself" (Matthew 22:37, 39). Similarly, Paul urges the Corinthians to reciprocate love freely: "We have spoken freely to you, Corinthians, and opened wide our hearts to you. We are not withholding our affection from you, but you are withholding yours from us... Open wide your hearts also" (2 Corinthians 6:11-13).

Just as our physical heart requires both an inflow and outflow of lifeblood, our loving heart, too, functions best when engaged in both giving and receiving. It is akin to a muscle, a trust muscle, which necessitates use and exercise to maintain strength. Failure to nurture this trust muscle can result in its injury, leading to diminished capacity to love.

Taking ownership of our ability to love is imperative. Concealing or rejecting love, whether consciously or subconsciously, can be detrimental to our well-being. Often, individuals deflect responsibility for their lack of responsiveness to love, attributing their loneliness to an inability to receive love from others. This mindset negates personal agency and perpetuates a cycle of emotional disconnection. To break free, we must acknowledge our role in fostering or impeding love's expression and actively work to strengthen our capacity for love.

Navigating the intricacies of love and relationships requires conscientious attention to our boundaries. While caring for what lies within our boundaries is challenging, so too is respecting the boundaries of others. Setting and upholding boundaries demand effort and vigilance, but the rewards of healthier, more fulfilling relationships are well worth the labor. As we explore in the following chapter, understanding and addressing boundary issues is essential for fostering greater relational harmony and personal growth.

Boundary Problems

Compliant: Saying Yes to the Bad

When parents teach children that setting boundaries or saying no is bad, they are teaching them that others can do with them as they wish. They are sending their children defenseless into a world that contains much evil: evil in the form of controlling, manipulative, and exploitative people, and evil in the form of temptations. To feel safe in such an evil world, children need to have the power to say things like: "No," "I disagree," "I will not," "I choose not to," "Stop that," "It hurts," "It's wrong," "That's bad," "I don't like it when you touch me there."

Blocking a child's ability to say no handicaps that child for life. Adults with handicaps like these experience their first boundary injury when they say yes to bad things. This type of boundary conflict is called compliance. Compliant people have fuzzy and indistinct boundaries; they "melt" into the demands and needs of other people. They can't stand alone, distinct from people who want something from them. Compliants, for example, pretend to like the same restaurants and movies their friends do "just to belong." They minimize their differences with others so as not to rock the boat. Compliants are chameleons. After a while, it's hard to distinguish them from their environment. The inability to say no to bad is pervasive. Not only does it keep us from refusing evil in our lives, it often keeps us from recognizing evil. Many compliant people realize too late that they're in a dangerous or abusive relationship. Their spiritual and emotional "radar" is broken; they have no ability to guard their hearts (Prov. 4:23).

This type of boundary problem paralyzes people's "no" muscles. Whenever they need to protect themselves by saying no, the word catches in their throats. This happens for a number of different reasons: fear of hurting the other person's feelings, fear of abandonment and separateness, a wish to be totally dependent on another, fear of someone else's anger, fear of punishment, fear of being ashamed, fear of being seen as bad or selfish, fear of being unspiritual, fear of one's overstrict, critical conscience.

This last fear is actually experienced as guilt. People who have an overstrict, critical conscience will condemn themselves for things God himself doesn't condemn them for. As Paul says, "Since their conscience is weak, it is defiled" (1 Cor. 8:7). Afraid to confront their unbiblical and critical internal parent, they tighten appropriate boundaries. When we give in to guilty feelings, we are complying with a harsh conscience. This fear of disobeying the harsh conscience translates into an inability to confront others—a saying yes to the bad—because it would cause more guilt.

Avoidants: Saying No to the good

Rachel had been the driving force behind the formation of the Bible study. She and her husband, Joe, had developed the format, invited the other couples, and opened up their homes to the study. Caught up in her leadership role, however, Rachel never opened up about her struggles. She shied away from such opportunities, preferring instead to help draw out others. Tonight, the others waited.

Rachel cleared her throat. Looking around the room, she finally spoke, "After hearing all the other problems in the room, I think the Lord's speaking to me. He seems to be saying that my issues are nothing compared to what you all deal with. It would be selfish to take up time with the little struggles I face. So... who'd like dessert?" No one spoke. But disappointment was evident on each face. Rachel had again avoided an opportunity for others to love her as they'd been loved by her.

This boundary problem is called avoidance: saying no to the good. It's the inability to ask for help, to recognize one's own need to let others in. Avoidants withdraw when they are in need; they do not ask for support from others.

Why is avoidance a boundary problem? At the heart of the struggle is the confusion of boundaries as walls. Boundaries are supposed to be able to "breathe," to be like fences with a gate that can let the good and the bad out. Individuals with walls for boundaries can let in neither bad nor good. No one touched them. God designed our personal boundaries to have gates. We should have the freedom to enjoy safe relationships and to avoid destructive ones. God even allows us the freedom to let him in or close him off: "Here I am! I stand at the door and knock. If anyone hears my voice and opens the door, I will come in and eat with him, and be with me" (Rev. 3:20).

God has no interest in violating our boundaries so that he can relate to us. He understands that this would cause injuries of trust. It is our responsibility to open up to him in need and repentance. Yet, for avoidants, opening up to both God and people is almost impossible.

The impermeable boundaries of avoidants cause a rigidity toward their God-given needs. They experience their problems and legitimate wants as something bad, destructive, or shameful.

Some people, like Marti, are both compliant and avoidant. In a recent session, Marti laughed ruefully at herself. "I'm beginning to see a pattern here. When someone needs four hours with me, I can't say no. I need someone for ten minutes, I can't ask for it. Isn't there a transistor in my head that I can replace?

Marti's dilemma is shared by many adults. She says "yes" to the bad (compliant) and says "no" to the good (avoidant). Individuals who have both boundary conflicts not only cannot refuse evil, they are unable to receive support they so readily offer to others. They are stuck in a cycle of feeling drained, but with nothing to replace lost energy. Compliant-avoidants suffer from what is called "reverse boundaries". They have no boundaries where they need them, and they have boundaries where they shouldn't have them.

Controllers: Not Respecting Others' Boundaries

"What do you mean, you're quitting? You can't leave now!" Steve looked across his desk at his administrative assistant. Frank had been working for Steve for several years and was finally fed up. He had given his all to the position, but Steve didn't know when to back off.

Time after time, Steve would insist on Frank spending unpaid time at the office on important projects. Frank had even switched his vacation schedule twice at Steve's insistence. But the final straw was when Steve began calling Frank at home. An occasional call at home Frank could understand. But almost every day, during dinner time, the family would wait while Frank had a telephone conference with his boss.

Several times Frank had tried to talk with Steve about the time violations. But Steve never really understood how burned out Frank was. After all, he needed Frank. Frank made him look successful. And it was easy to get him to work harder.

Steve has a problem hearing and accepting others' boundaries. To Steve, no is simply a challenge to change the other person's mind. This boundary problem is control. Controllers can't respect others' limits. They resist taking responsibility for their own lives, so they need to control others.

Controllers believe the old jokes about training top salespeople: no means maybe and maybe means yes. While this may be productive in learning to sell a product, it can wreak havoc in a relationship. Controllers are perceived as bullies, manipulative, and aggressive.

The primary problem of individuals who can't hear no—which is different from not being able to say no—is that they project responsibility for their lives onto others. They use various means of control to motivate others to carry the load intended by God to be theirs alone.

Remember the "boulder and knapsack" illustration in chapter 2? Controllers look for someone to carry their knapsacks (individual responsibilities) in addition to their boulders (crises and crushing burdens). Had Steve shouldered the weight of his own job, Frank would have been happy to pitch in extra hours from time to time. But the pressure of covering for Steve's irresponsibility made a talented professional look elsewhere for work.

Controllers come in two types:

Aggressive controllers are individuals who clearly disregard others' boundaries. They bulldoze over people's fences like a tank, sometimes resorting to verbal or even physical abuse. However, most of the time, they are simply oblivious to the existence of boundaries. It's as if they live in a world where only "yes" matters, with no room for someone else's "no." They relentlessly try to force others to conform to their own ideas of how life should be, neglecting their own responsibility to accept others as they are.

An example of an aggressive controller is Peter. When Jesus was explaining to the disciples about his upcoming suffering, death, and resurrection, Peter took it upon himself to rebuke Jesus. In response, Jesus rebuked Peter, saying, "Get behind me, Satan! You do not have in mind the things of God, but the things of men" (Mark 8:33). Peter's refusal to accept the Lord's boundaries prompted an immediate confrontation from Jesus.

Manipulative controllers, on the other hand, are less overt than aggressive controllers. They employ tactics to persuade others to disregard their boundaries, coaxing them into saying "yes" when they should say "no." They manipulate circumstances indirectly to achieve their desired outcomes and often use guilt as a tool.

A classic example of manipulation is seen in Tom Sawyer, who tricked his friends into whitewashing the fence for him, making it seem like a privilege. Similarly, Jacob, the son of Isaac, manipulated his twin brother Esau into giving up his birthright and deceived his father to receive Esau's blessing (Genesis 25:29-34; 27:1-29). Jacob's very name means "deceiver," and he frequently used his cunning to circumvent others' boundaries.

However, Jacob's encounter with God in human form marked a turning point in his life. During a night-long struggle with God, Jacob wrestled with his own deceitfulness. God ultimately changed Jacob's name to Israel, meaning "he who fights with God." This event symbolized Jacob's transformation from a manipulative deceiver to a more honest individual. He began to own his assertiveness, evident in his new name. Similarly, only when a manipulative controller is confronted with their dishonesty can they take responsibility for their actions, repent, and accept both their own and others' boundaries.

CHAPTER 6: SEEK CLARITY

Our research unequivocally demonstrates that high performers possess a distinct advantage over their peers: they exude clarity. They know precisely who they are, what they want, how to attain it, and what brings them genuine fulfillment. Interestingly, enhancing someone's clarity invariably elevates their overall performance metrics.

Now, if you're sitting there wondering whether you possess such clarity, fear not. It's not an inherent trait reserved for a select few. Think of clarity like electricity in a power plant—it's not something you either have or don't have; rather, it's something you generate and harness. So, waiting for a sudden epiphany to illuminate your path forward isn't the answer. Instead, clarity is cultivated through inquiry, exploration, experimentation, and thoughtful introspection.

Successful individuals, we've discovered, have a firm grasp on fundamental questions: Who am I? What do I value? What are my strengths and weaknesses? What are my goals, and what's my plan to achieve them? These seemingly elementary inquiries wield immense influence over one's life trajectory.

Clarity regarding self-identity correlates strongly with self-esteem, while its absence aligns with neuroticism and negative emotions. Self-awareness lays the foundation for initial success. Knowing oneself breeds confidence and direction, essential elements for navigating life's complexities.

Furthermore, setting clear and challenging goals, backed by specific deadlines and actionable plans, is paramount. Research spanning decades underscores the potency of specific, ambitious objectives in driving performance and satisfaction. Goals serve as beacons, propelling us toward greater productivity and fulfillment.

But goals without deadlines and plans are mere wishes, susceptible to the whims of procrastination and distraction. Establishing concrete timelines and detailed action plans significantly enhances the likelihood of goal attainment, even on days when motivation wanes.

Remember, clarity of vision begets clarity of life. Embrace the power of the written word; jot down your thoughts, ambitions, and strategies. As the adage goes, "The shortest pencil is better than the longest memory." Don't squander your most precious asset—time—by deferring action. Seize the present moment and commit to clarity.

So, read, pause, and write. Embrace the journey, irrespective of your past. Your history doesn't dictate your destiny. Let go of yesterday's limitations and focus on crafting a compelling future. The time for clarity is now.

The Top 3%

Why is today so monumental? Because today marks your commitment to manifesting your aspirations by putting pen to paper. Allow me to share a staggering revelation: Dr. Gale Matthews conducted a study revealing that the simple act of jotting down your goals increases your likelihood of achieving them by a whopping 42%.

Yes, you read that right. Merely writing down your goals propels you nearly halfway toward their realization! So, seize that paper and pen—no, not your computer; embrace the tangible act of handwriting. It's a mental pledge, a subtle yet profound commitment to your dreams. Remember, it's the small adjustments that yield monumental achievements—the peaks that beckon you to ascend.

Consider this: a staggering 97% of Americans bypass the transformative power of written goals. By committing your aspirations to paper, you catapult yourself into the esteemed 3%, poised to navigate an elevated realm of achievement.

Now, let's dispel any notion that success is exclusive to Ivy League elites. Take Harvard Business School, for instance. In a comprehensive study tracking its alumni's trajectories, a remarkable pattern emerged: the top echelon of achievers—all boasting unparalleled power, influence, and financial success—shared a common denominator: they had documented goals. Conversely, those who neglected this practice failed to sustain their momentum, despite their prestigious pedigrees.

Intriguingly, within the same cohort, researchers uncovered a poignant reality: despite their academic accolades and networks, three Harvard graduates found themselves employed yet homeless. Their poignant narrative underscores the critical distinction between mere credentials and the transformative power of intentional goal setting.

So, as you embark on this journey of clarity and purpose, remember: the act of writing your goals isn't just a task; it's a catalyst for extraordinary achievement. Embrace the power of intention, and let your written aspirations pave the path to unparalleled success.

You're in Good Company

Imagine a company akin to the brilliance of Will Smith. Picture this: a narrative unfolds of an individual granted entry into Will's abode. Upon crossing the threshold, he finds himself ensconced within a sprawling, opulent residence adorned with glass walls. Yet, the view beyond is obscured by an array of meticulously placed paper fragments.

Puzzled, the visitor inquires, "What are these?" Will, with a knowing smile, gestures towards the scattered notes. "Ah, those," he replies, "that's my latest project—a movie in the making." To the untrained eye, it appears chaotic, far from the polished image of a cinematic masterpiece. But to Will, it's a canvas awaiting transformation.

With an air of excitement, Will embarks on a guided tour of his creative process. He expounds on the importance of well-crafted characters, the essential presence of antagonists, and the art of concealing the journey's conclusion to deliver a compelling plot twist. He stresses the significance of emotional depth, the ebb and flow of highs and lows, all woven seamlessly into a captivating storyline.

His guest, initially bewildered by the complexity, finds himself overwhelmed, massaging his temples in an attempt to digest the wealth of information. Sensing his apprehension, Will reassures him with a grin, "It's simpler than you think. Start with the end in mind—the goal—and chart your course backward."

Indeed, Will Smith approaches each cinematic endeavor with a clear endpoint in sight: the culmination of his vision. Similarly, what you commit to paper today is not merely a goal; it's the genesis of your narrative—the blueprint for your journey to success.

In the words of Zig Ziglar, "A goal properly set is halfway reached." So, let your aspirations guide you, and may your story unfold with purpose and determination.

A Goal is Like a Destination

Imagine I called you right now, breathless with excitement, and invited you on a spontaneous road trip. Picture me promising to swing by your place in just 15 minutes to whisk you away. Naturally, your first question would be: "Where are we headed?" You'd need to know how to pack—are we bound for snowy peaks, sunny shores, or perhaps a thought-provoking conference?

Now, let's imagine we hit the road with no destination in mind, spending a whole hour debating our route. Eventually, we settle on a beach day, but by then, we've already sped 80 mph in the wrong direction, hurtling toward Kansas. We've wasted precious time and energy, ill-prepared for the adventure ahead with all the wrong gear packed.

This scenario mirrors what occurs when we lack a clear goal in life. Without a destination, we meander aimlessly, squandering valuable resources and arriving unprepared for what awaits us. We must chart our course with precision; there's no room for small plans here.

So, let's embark on this journey of dreams, where the magnitude of our aspirations should stir a hint of trepidation. Our potential is vast—far greater than we realize. The pace is about to quicken, and the stakes are high. Are you ready? Do you have your pen and paper at the ready, your imagination fueled, and your dreams ready to take flight? Excellent. It's time to inscribe your goals onto the canvas of your future.

To guide you on this transformative path, here are a few principles to illuminate your way forward:

Step 1: Limit Your Goals to 7-10

Why? Well, in the past, I've fallen into the trap of setting too many goals—10 spiritual ones, 10 financial aspirations, 10 personal targets, and the list goes on. But with each goal I added, I found myself spreading thin, chasing too many rabbits, and ultimately, achieving less than I aimed for. It left me feeling defeated rather than accomplished.

Studies confirm this phenomenon. Dividing our focus among numerous goals often leads to missed targets and a loss of momentum. There's wisdom in the saying, "If you chase too many rabbits, you won't catch any of them." Research suggests that setting seven to ten goals allows us to concentrate our efforts and pursue what truly matters to us.

Write Your Goals Swiftly

Research also indicates that we should spend no more than three minutes jotting down our goals. Any longer, and we risk talking ourselves out of them. Doubts creep in: "That's too ambitious for me," or "I'm not sure I can pull that off." Three minutes is all it takes—no excuses.

So, seize this moment. While the questions still linger in your mind—what would make this year extraordinary? Are you aligned with God's plan?—write down your goals. Be bold. No one will see them but you. Feel the power of seeing your aspirations materialize on paper. Does it stir excitement? Does it provoke a bit of fear? Or perhaps, is there a deep sense of peace, even in the face of challenges?

Write in the Present Tense

Now, let's refine our approach:

- Limit your goals to 7-10.
- Write them swiftly.
- And now, write them in the present tense.

As 2 Corinthians 5:7 reminds us, "We walk by faith and not by sight." We're speaking words of faith, envisioning our goals as accomplished realities. We're not merely hoping; we're declaring with confidence. So, pen your goals as if they've already come to fruition: "I am at my perfect weight." "I reside in a mortgage-free home." "I have secured admission to..." "I have attained the promotion, bearing the title of..."

Write them down, for they are the roadmap to your future success.

"Who do you think you are?" It's a question that echoes through the corridors of doubt when the journey gets tough, when uncertainty looms large. In those moments, we must stand firm, anchoring ourselves to our goals and declaring them as if they're already accomplished. Just as Jesus faced temptation in Matthew 4, challenged by the adversary, we too will encounter obstacles on the path to our dreams.

The enemy's whispers will insidiously probe our resolve: "Why do you think you have the right? Who do you think you are?" Yet, like Jesus, our response must remain unwavering, echoing the same resolute affirmation: "It is written."

With our goals firmly entrenched in our minds and hearts, we can boldly proclaim to the adversary, "This is my vision. I've consulted with the Divine, and this is my ordained path. I know my identity. I belong to the Most High, and I serve the Provider, my Father. When you challenge me, you challenge the forces of heaven."

Knowing our identity—knowing whose we are—is paramount. We must engrave our vision upon the tablet of our consciousness, keeping it ever before us as a guiding light. When the enemy seeks to sow doubt, we stand firm in our truth.

The cycle of dissatisfaction can be broken. We hold the power to pivot, to refine, to reach higher. It begins with the simple act of writing our goals with conviction, as if preparing to set them into motion.

So, let us rewrite the narrative of our lives. Let us embrace intentionality, turning our aspirations into concrete plans. With clarity of purpose and steadfast faith, we pave the way for a future defined by accomplishment and fulfillment.

***

Be Specific: The Power of Clarity

Clarity of vision begets clarity of life—it's a truth that has shaped the trajectories of countless success stories, including that of Oprah Winfrey. Oprah didn't just dream of becoming wealthy; she had a crystal-clear vision of her goals. At the tender age of 19, she declared with unwavering conviction that she would be a millionaire by 32, not a year earlier or later. Moreover, she aspired to be the richest black woman in America. With pinpoint precision, she mapped out her path, setting a specific age and position for her achievements. And true to her vision, nineteen years later, Oprah stood exactly where she had envisioned—right on schedule.

There's a profound distinction between a mere resolution and a concrete goal. As you embark on this journey of goal-setting, remember to be specific. You're not simply jotting down vague aspirations to be forgotten in the labyrinth of your thoughts. No, you're committing your dreams to paper, infusing them with clarity and focus.

Consider, for instance, a desire to work with animals. What does that entail? Are you drawn to veterinary medicine, animal conservation, or perhaps animal welfare advocacy? This is your opportunity to delineate your path, to carve out a clear direction for your aspirations. Write swiftly, within three minutes, capturing the essence of your dreams in precise detail.

For clarity isn't just a human concept—it's a divine mandate. Habakkuk 2:2 implores us to inscribe our visions upon tablets, to articulate them plainly for all to see. So, write down your goals where you can see them, and be specific. Say it aloud: "I'm going to be specific." Let the resonance of your words affirm your commitment to precision.

In the realm of sales, precision reigns supreme. Studies have shown that the more specific our requests, the higher the likelihood of a positive response. From asking for spare change to soliciting a specific amount, the power of specificity is undeniable. And this principle extends to our personal goals—the clearer we are with ourselves, the more responsive we become to our aspirations.

As Bill Copeland astutely observed, "The trouble with not having a goal is that you can spend your life running up and down the field and never score." So, let us not wander aimlessly but chart our course with clarity and intentionality. By embracing specificity, we unlock the door to a future defined by achievement and fulfillment.

Step Two: Turn Your Goals Into Vision

A solitary thought, much like a lone raindrop, lacks the power to nurture a flourishing garden. Merely contemplating your goals once, then walking away, is akin to that lone raindrop. Yet, when thoughts multiply—when compelling mental images, steeped in emotion, result from the continuous contemplation and review of your goals—a synergy is born. Like a deluge of rain, these thoughts saturate and nourish the soil from which your dreams will blossom.

The beauty of this process lies in its innate alignment with your essence. These dreams, these goals—they are yours by birthright. Now, you're poised to elevate them to the next level, to traverse the path toward manifesting your dreams. You're embarking on the most rewarding investment of your life. As Warren Buffet aptly remarked, "When you invest in yourself, you get a 1,000% return."

Clarity of vision begets clarity of life. Have you truly seen what you desire out of life? If not, perhaps it's because clarity has eluded you. Visualization holds the key to transforming your goals into vivid, internalized visions.

Visualization isn't a novel concept—it's a tool wielded by the most successful salespeople. Picture yourself in a new car showroom, engrossed in conversation with a salesperson. "Can you envision yourself driving this car?" they inquire. Eventually, you nod in agreement, "Yes, I can see myself driving this car." Suddenly, a car that was once invisible to you now dominates your field of vision.

The power of visualization lies in its ability to bridge the gap between possibility and reality, shifting our perception from the confines of our minds to the tangible world around us. Soon enough, you'll find yourself watching others drive down the street in your dream car, spurred on by the fervent desire to make it your own.

Years ago, there was a man driving with friends in Hawaii. They saw the home of the late Elvis Presley. The driver said to his friend, "Can you imagine living in a house like that?"

The other man replied, "No, I sure can't."

The first man, a successful man, said, "And you never will, because you cannot be what you cannot see!"

Your subconscious mind has the ability to steer your life toward your dreams through the power of visualization. Become the person who can envision the future with great clarity! You have to see it to be it! What are you ready to see right now?

Make your own vision board. Create one for home and one for work. Take a picture of it and set it as the screensaver on your phone. Envision yourself in these places through the lens of faith on your vision board. Then, one day, you'll believe it so deeply that you can see your future clearly without it.

Step Three: Get Going

Follow a MAP! If we don't have a destination in mind, we won't know how to plot the course, and we'll never know when we get there.

The "M" in MAP is for Measure. You have to know where you are so that you can mark your progress. There are a lot of things we can measure in life - our health, wealth, emotional and mental well-being, and dreams.

The "A" in MAP stands for Assess. We need to assess where we are today so that we can develop an action plan by asking: How are we going to do that? If you are going to write a book, you have to start writing something - anything! When? When are you going to start writing? Where? Do you have a certain place where you want to write? How? How will you write? Will you use a special notebook? A computer? An app? What? What are you going to write? It does not have to be big. You can write a blog, journal every day, or research and write a first draft of a book proposal. It all starts with assessing and asking the right questions that will lead to an action plan.

Where Focus Goes, Energy Flows. Asking questions will start energy flowing in the direction of your dreams.

"P" is for Plan. Once you decide what you need to do and the order you need to do it in, you can begin to see things happen in your life. You can't go anywhere without a plan. Goals without plans are just dreams, and dreams are hard to remember when you wake up.

Step 4: Get Results

Transitioning from initiation to achievement marks this step. While motivation kick-starts the journey, commitment ensures the delivery of results.

Every day, consciously or unconsciously, we are shaping our habits. Unintentionally, we might find ourselves hitting the snooze button repeatedly, moving sluggishly, relying on that first cup of coffee to jumpstart our day, and rushing through traffic due to tardiness. Alternatively, we can choose to live with purposeful intent.

Successful individuals distinguish themselves by making the tough choices that yield delayed gratification. They persevere where others falter, embracing failure as a stepping stone to success. They refuse to succumb to adversity, persisting until they reach their breakthrough moment. The path to success often entails traversing numerous unsuccessful routes before uncovering the one that leads to triumph.

Focus

Distractions often hinder our progress towards achieving our goals. It's crucial to have the ability to refocus when life becomes chaotic. When things get blurry, adjust your focus accordingly. Time may be limited, and unexpected urgencies such as illness, significant projects, relationship stress, or boredom may arise. In such moments, we face a choice: give up or rise to the occasion.

Setbacks are inevitable. You may encounter failures, experience weight gain, overspend, or lose your temper. However, instead of letting these challenges derail you, commit to failing forward – using setbacks as stepping stones toward success. This approach equips you with valuable insights, ensuring you know exactly how to navigate future obstacles.

It's often the unnoticed small actions that yield the desired results. Discipline serves as the bridge between your aspirations and your accomplishments, narrowing the gap between who you are and who you strive to become.

Execution: The Good Kind

Executing your plans means pushing through when it's easy and refusing to quit when faced with challenges. It's about committing to the grind, even when the going gets tough. Let's be real – execution is work. It's rolling up your sleeves and getting things done, staying focused amidst distractions. It's where intentions meet action, where dreams meet reality.

The adversary may try to derail us with countless distractions, but remember, he can't destroy our path unless we allow him to. We must remain steadfast in our commitment to execution, unwavering in the face of adversity.

God calls us to be strong and courageous not because the journey will be easy, but because faith is integral to success. Along the way, there will be temptations to step aside, to let someone else take the reins of our destiny while we sit on the sidelines. But the key to victory lies in perseverance – in relentlessly putting one foot in front of the other, even when victory seems uncertain. The surefire way to lose is to quit.

By cultivating faith-filled thoughts and speaking words of belief, we empower ourselves to translate our aspirations into tangible actions. It's through execution – where faith transforms into action – that we bring to life the dreams, visions, businesses, callings, and plans that have been placed within us. God waits for us to do our part before unleashing His full power. To maximize the divine investment in us – His love, His Son, our talents, and purpose – we must fully commit to execution.

As the legendary coach Vince Lombardi once said, "You'll either have reasons or you'll have results. Which one do you want?"

Forge the Right Circle of Friends:

Where the Right People Lead to the Right Results

Our goals aren't merely about reaching the destination; they're about sustaining our progress. Day by day, inch by inch, step by step, we embark on a journey of listening, learning, improving, and growing in knowledge, strength, and character.

Be cautious about sharing your aspirations with those who seek to undermine your ambitions. Instead, confide in individuals who refuse to let you falter when faced with adversity – those who uplift you, believe in you, and pray for your success. Seek out trustworthy companions who will hold you accountable, whether in moments of joy or when the path ahead feels arduous. Purposefully seek at least one person who not only celebrates your achievements but also challenges you to aim higher. Surround yourself with groups of individuals who inspire you and refine your skills. This process is more vital than you may realize.

Remember, the company we keep can profoundly influence our journey towards success. Choose your circle wisely, for the right people will not only support you but also propel you towards the right results.

Step 5: Get Rest

Perhaps you're not meant to throw in the towel just yet. Maybe what you truly need is a break – a well-deserved pause in your journey thus far. Consider it a small reward for your hard work. You might be thinking, "I don't have time to rest." But in all honesty, you can't afford not to.

Rest isn't merely idle time; it's an opportunity to sharpen your tools. Ever heard the tale of the two lumberjacks vying for the same job? One worked tirelessly without breaks, while the other took intermittent pauses to sharpen his axe. Despite initial assumptions, it was the latter who emerged as the victor. Why? Because he understood the importance of rejuvenation and preparation.

Similarly, rest rejuvenates not only our bodies but also our souls. It's a chance to relinquish control and trust in a higher power. Often, we overestimate our ability to manage situations and underestimate divine intervention. It's time to distinguish between good ideas and God's plans. Surrender the burden of worry and allow yourself the luxury of peace.

Even though we acknowledge the necessity of rest, many of us struggle to grant ourselves permission to indulge in it fully. Doubt, worry, and guilt plague our minds. But remember, taking care of yourself isn't selfish; it's essential for your well-being and effectiveness in the long run.

So, make rest a priority. Release the weight of responsibility and trust that everything will fall into place. Start small, and gradually entrust larger concerns to a higher power. It's time to let go of the need to control every outcome and embrace the restorative power of surrender.

Rest To Renewal

Stop resisting. God requires your unique talents, but He also demands your well-being. To serve at your best, you must prioritize rest; otherwise, you risk burning out and becoming ineffective. Recognize that the doubts and fears whispering in your mind are merely tactics of the enemy, seeking to rob you of the rest you desperately need.

Rest doesn't have to be elusive. There are numerous natural methods to enhance your ability to rest. Start by establishing boundaries – designate a specific hour to stop working, turn off your phone, and resist the temptation to check emails. Instead, engage in activities that soothe your mind and spirit. Whether it's taking a leisurely stroll, immersing yourself in a good book, or enjoying quality time with loved ones, find what brings you joy and peace.

Simple gestures can also aid in relaxation. Consider incorporating lavender oil on your pillowcase or trying supplements like magnesium or melatonin (after consulting with your healthcare provider). Invest in comfortable bedding and establish a bedtime routine that signals to your mind it's time to unwind.

Indulge in self-care rituals such as aromatic baths or showers with soothing salts. Dim the lights, read a devotional or a few passages from the Bible, and express gratitude for the blessings of the day. These practices help prepare your mind, body, and spirit for a restful night's sleep.

Don't underestimate the power of rest in rejuvenating your soul and enhancing your productivity. Embrace the journey towards replenishment, and allow yourself to experience the transformative power of surrendering to rest.

Unlock Your Rewards

Why do we often neglect this crucial step? It's essential to celebrate every milestone on the journey to your ultimate destination. Without acknowledgment and appreciation of your progress, the path ahead may seem daunting, discouraging, and endless, leading you to contemplate giving up.

Take a moment to recognize where you are right now. You've diligently planned and pursued your goals. Now, it's time to reap the rewards of your hard work. Remember, "God will grant you the desires of your heart" and ensure the success of your endeavors. As you strive for your ambitions, don't forget to assess whether you're also evolving into the person you aspire to be in all aspects of your life.

The true value of achieving your goals lies not only in the tangible rewards but also in the personal growth you experience along the way.

Small victories can have a big impact.

Rewards come in various shapes and sizes. Sometimes, they manifest as small rays of sunshine that illuminate our days. These rewards need not come with a hefty price tag. Whether it's a moment of solitude, a leisurely stroll, or a simple indulgence, take time to celebrate the victories, no matter how small, on your journey to victory.

Consider what these rewards mean to you personally. What victories do you wish to commemorate, and where along your path can you plan these celebrations? Deliberately scheduling these moments of joy and acknowledgment will infuse your journey with happiness, enthusiasm, and momentum. The key is to plan them intentionally, to define what triumph looks like for you, and to revel in each step forward.

So, as you pursue your goals, remember to pause, celebrate, and cherish the victories, both big and small, that pave the way to your ultimate success.

CHAPTER 7:
THE POWER OF HAPPINESS

Happiness Habit 1: Define & Feel What Happiness Looks Like To YOU

Picture us seated in a cozy restaurant, the air alive with anticipation. Now, imagine I pose a question that delves deep into your soul: "What truly makes you happy?" Would you have an immediate answer? It's a question that stirs contemplation, for often, we struggle to articulate our personal definition of happiness. Why? Because we're accustomed to comparing our aspirations to those of others, allowing their desires to overshadow our own.

Take a moment now to reflect or jot down your thoughts on what ignites your heart, brightens your eyes, and fills you with boundless joy. Think back to your childhood or earlier years – when did you feel most at peace, most alive? Was it the thrill of a sporting event, the tranquility of fishing, or the serenity of the ocean's embrace?

Now, consider your present-day sources of happiness. What delights your soul in this moment? Remember, your list may evolve over time. What once brought you joy may hold less significance now, replaced by newfound passions and experiences.

It's crucial to differentiate between happiness and goals. While we may pursue materialistic or achievement-oriented objectives, true happiness transcends these ambitions. Take a moment to discern the distinction between your aspirations and the fundamental sources of your happiness.

Begin your journey toward happiness by defining what it means to you in your current life. Start by jotting down your thoughts without overanalyzing them. Include not only activities that bring you joy but also thoughts that uplift your spirit and blessings you're grateful for. Write freely, allowing your heart to guide the way.

Once you've compiled your list, revisit it and identify three to five items that resonate deeply with you. These are your pillars of happiness, your guiding lights on the path to joy. Embrace them, cherish them, and allow them to lead you toward a life filled with authentic happiness.

Happiness Habit 2: Befriend Your Present

When we speak of making the present your friend, we're not referring to the gifts under the Christmas tree. We're talking about embracing the here and now – this very moment you're experiencing. It's about forging a friendship with the present rather than constantly yearning for tomorrow, next week, or next year. How often do we find ourselves fixated on the future, believing that happiness awaits us only when certain conditions are met? We say to ourselves, "When I achieve this milestone, then I'll be happy." But this kind of thinking is a mere postponement of joy, a perpetual deferral to an uncertain future.

Consider how often you catch yourself dwelling on the future, caught in a cycle of "when/then" scenarios. "When I reach this goal, then I'll feel content." By fixating on an elusive future, we overlook the beauty and potential for happiness in the present moment. What if we chose to be happy right now, in this very second? What if we stopped dwelling on the past and fretting about the future, and instead focused on cultivating joy and gratitude in the present?

It's easy to get caught up in the cycle of future-focused thinking, anticipating what might go wrong and overlooking the blessings of today. But the key to inner peace and happiness lies in embracing the present moment. As Eckhart Tolle eloquently states in "The Power of Now," true contentment is found when we live fully in the present.

Let go of the past, release your grip on the future, and seize the gift of the present with both hands. Embrace the opportunities, appreciate your health and vitality, and relish the simple pleasures of life. Remember, happiness isn't a destination to be reached; it's a choice to be made in every moment. So, why wait? Choose happiness today.

Happiness Habit 3: Free Yourself From Overthinking

Ever heard of the saying, "Paralysis caused by over-analysis"? It's a phenomenon that plagues many of us, halting our progress and preventing us from living the life we truly desire. I've witnessed this pattern unfold time and again, particularly when individuals are on the cusp of embarking on new ventures or reaching for greater heights in their careers and wealth. What holds them back? Simply put, it's overthinking.

No matter the goal or aspiration, overthinking can be the silent saboteur of progress. It's the relentless cycle of analysis paralysis that leaves us stagnant and stuck in indecision. I've seen singles yearning for love talk themselves out of potential relationships with a barrage of "what ifs" and hypothetical scenarios. "Should I pursue this connection? What if it doesn't work out? What if we have different beliefs?" Before they know it, they've talked themselves out of taking a chance, potentially missing out on a meaningful connection.

It's essential to gather the necessary knowledge and information to build confidence in your decisions. However, there comes a point where endless questioning and circular analysis become counterproductive. When your heart whispers, urging you to take action, and your subconscious nudges you forward, it's time to silence the overthinking and seize the moment.

Instead of getting lost in a maze of doubts and uncertainties, trust your instincts and intuition. Embrace the courage to step outside your comfort zone and take decisive action. Remember, happiness often lies on the other side of fear and hesitation. So, break free from the shackles of overthinking, and start moving towards your dreams with confidence and conviction.

Happiness Habit 4: Focus on A Positive Outcome

This is a powerful way to bring happiness into your life and get what you want in advance. And I know it sounds simple, but I can't tell you how many times I've heard someone say, "Oh Dean, you're too optimistic." Am I too optimistic or do I just understand how powerful our subconscious is? Listen, your energy is going to go in any direction you aim it; you get to choose if it is spent on the positive or the negative. I know so many people who focus on what could go wrong in life rather than what could go right. One day they may feel a little run down and they conjure worst-case scenarios: "What if this is really me getting sick? What if it's the flu, I never got the flu shot? What if I have an illness that could kill me? I don't have health insurance, man I am in trouble!" Guess what? People like this will talk themselves right into getting sick! Why not put all the energy into focusing on a positive outcome and perfect health and more wealth, happiness, and abundance? Concentrate on thoughts of good health and a long life.

Consider the results of studies about driving on long roads with only one tree: Most, if not all, accidents on these roads involve someone running into that one tree. Because people may be rushing through traffic or lose control of the wheel and think to themselves, "I don't want to hit that tree. I don't want to hit a tree. I don't want to hit that tree." And what do they do? They hit the darn tree.

The world has programmed us to think a certain way about situations we face. When something comes up, our minds immediately want to go, "Oh no, this isn't good! What if, what if." The antidote: Become a keen observer of your thoughts. It worked for me. And now, when what-if thoughts try to sneak into my mind I say, "No, no, no. I'm not going to let my mind go there." Yes, I could focus on the negative and be stressed and worried about what could happen, but I decided years ago that I was no longer going to do that. You can focus on what might go wrong or you can focus on what might go right. Why not invest your energy in what can go right?

I used to focus on the wrong outcomes, and this story from my own personal hell illustrates the dangers of this focus. For years, I woke up at 2:00 in the morning because my mind was racing with thoughts. And for years I just thought this early morning waking was a reason for my success. I'd wake up and I'd start thinking about things going on that day and I'd think about what could go wrong and I'd try to find solutions to them before the problems even were reality! Half the time I wouldn't be able to fall back asleep because I would get obsessed with these imaginary bad outcomes and become stressed. Then one day, I said to myself, "No more! I'm going to start tricking my mind and my subconscious by changing those negative thoughts I wake up with. From now on I'm only going to focus on a positive outcome to these situations rather than creating negative outcomes in my mind." And what happened? I was able to visualize success and happiness and finally started getting much-needed sleep. It took some time to make the transition from negative to positive outcomes, but when I replaced that disempowering habit with the empowering habit, it eventually stuck.

Trent Shelton is a former NFL player who is the founder of Rehab Time where each week through social media he delivers powerful, inspirational, and uplifting messages. Trent has transcended his career as a football player to become an amazing motivational speaker and inspirational leader. He may have been in the spotlight as a football player, but he has a much more visible and prominent role now as millions of people see his videos and posts each month.

He gets tens of thousands of positive, uplifting posts from people expressing their gratitude for his dedication to their greatness. With so much exposure, though, comes some negativity - the haters.

When I interviewed Trent, our conversations provided many great lessons, including his sharing his own Happiness Habit that helped him deal effectively with the pessimists and naysayers, both online and in his life. "First, I've come to associate a hateful post from someone as a disillusioned fan who is unconsciously still in need of some hope or motivation. It's so easy to scroll down and see a post under a video I sent out that can immediately affect my mindset. I'm human, just like everyone else. But when I simply gave that negative post a new meaning, it created a new behavior in me. No longer did I see it as I did something to create this; rather, I see it as, 'This person still needs help and hopefully, he will come around.' But I'm not in control of what I do. I let the tens of thousands of positive posts from the people who get inspired by my words be my fuel.

"And to protect myself even further I'm very picky about who I follow, what I do, what I watch, and honestly, even the conversations I have… I'm very selective about certain people when they call me because I know certain people either want something or they want to gossip or want to bring drama, so I always tell myself to protect my peace. So I will do what I must to put barricades between me and their negativity. Protect your peace every day and watch your happiness and joy grow.

"And I have another habit to start each day off the best I can. When I wake up, I put myself in the Championship Mode mindset, as I like to call it. I give thanks for the opportunity for life, for another day to give it my all. It's my biggest thing for protecting my confidence and protecting my peace because so many times, we don't realize the opportunity we have to give our greatness inside of us, and we can't share it and use it if we are not at peace. Do what you must to protect your peace and show the world what you are made of."

So be like Trent and don't let the naysayers in any area of your life bring you down. Switch it up and try to find how to give it a new meaning. "Protect your peace" are words Trent often uses, and so should you. In many cases, suffering is a choice. Therefore, do what you must, create new habits, and avoid suffering whenever possible. You are amazing; let the world see this incredible part of you every day.

Happiness Habit 5: Let Go of Specific Outcomes

This is a game changer. It's not easy, but it's damn effective. Too often, we predict what different outcomes should be and we get hung up on our predictions. "If I put this money into this deal, and I partner with this person, we should make x amount of money and here's exactly how it should look." Then if it doesn't turn out like that, happiness goes away. You think to yourself, "That's not what I wanted! That's not what I predicted! This isn't right! Sometimes you order steak, and the server brings you chicken and all of a sudden you're angry. 'This is not what I wanted! I can't believe this lie.'"

Here's how we make the same mistake in relationships: "We're going to be married next year and we're going to honeymoon in Hawaii, and this is the way it's going to be."

And when it doesn't turn out that way, we immediately get angry or our joy in the relationship diminishes.

Remember what Tony Robbins said: "What if life happens for us, not to us?" Imagine you're paddling downstream in a canoe and all of a sudden the current takes you off course. You could resist it and say, "I have to paddle upstream against this strong current and get back on the track I expected." But wouldn't that take a tremendous amount of effort? What if the course is altered, instead of being angry we said, "What if this little change in direction is a strategic part of my next level of life? Maybe this is happening for me and not to me. Maybe I should just ride the current out and see where it goes."

Many times when an entrepreneur starts a business, the original idea doesn't work. So the entrepreneur changes course and finds success in a totally unexpected direction. For example, that's how Twitter was born, almost by accident. Twitter started by its co-founders to be a podcast company where you could call a number to create a podcast. It wasn't even called Twitter. Then, iTunes announced that it was going to make podcasting available on all major Apple devices and suddenly Odeo (the company now known as Twitter) was in trouble! They had brainstorm meeting after brainstorm meeting to think of a new direction for the company and eventually came across the idea we all now know as Twitter! And that success would never have happened if the entrepreneurs had given up because their original concept didn't pan out.

When you're fixated on "riding the current" to one specific outcome, you become unhappy when things don't work out. When you're mired in unhappiness, you're never going to be successful. Instead, you lose confidence and walk around depressed. When you let go of a very specific outcome, the heavy weight of expectation comes off your shoulders. You will become a different person immediately, and your happiness will skyrocket.

Happiness Habit 6: Don't Be Afraid To Fail

We were raised to think that failure is bad. But truthfully, failure is the cornerstone of success. I'm looking at the quote on the wall right now by Winston Churchill, and it reads, "The definition of success is going from failure without losing your enthusiasm." When was the last time you embraced failure in your life?

Usually, if you're not failing, that means you're not pushing yourself hard enough and you're not trying new things. It means you're stuck in a rut and just going with the flow, or you're not straying from well-worn routines. But here's the thing: you'll never achieve anything on autopilot. So I say fail often and change the meaning of failure in your mind. I want you to be able to proudly say, "I failed today; I tried something new."

When you embrace failure, you will no longer feel sad when something doesn't go as planned. But what if you just got rid of that fearful attitude? When that happens, you replace your fear with an acceptance of changes in your life. Wayne Gretzky said it best, "You miss 100% of the shots you don't take." Embrace failure as a necessary part of success, and aim to do it daily.

Happiness Habit 7: Let Go Of Grudges

Another way of stating this habit is: Try not to take things personally. I know this is a tough one. But when you hold a grudge, you are holding that inside of you at the expense of your happiness, health, and success. Have you ever held a grudge against a parent, boss, relative, or somebody who did something horrible to you, and you obsess about it all the time? Just so you know, the grudge isn't affecting the offending party. As much as you boil and stew, your grudge-filled thoughts don't harm a hair on anyone's head. They do hurt you and your future success. You have to let go of all grudges, which I know is easier said than done.

When I let those grudges go, my happiness rose to a new level. Letting go of past grudges was one of the most liberating things I've ever done, and I urge you to take a look at your life and find the grudges you can release. If you do, you'll free yourself to be the best you possible.

Happiness Habit 8: Be Grateful For What's in Front of You

We all know that being grateful is the cornerstone of happiness. It's one of those things that you have to be consciously aware of daily. You could be struggling, need money, have debt or overdue bills, or going through a divorce, but there's always the opportunity to find gratitude for things in our lives.

I know life can be like a kick in the teeth sometimes. But gratitude can overcome anything, and the best way to start is by focusing on small things for which you're appreciative. You can be grateful for a smile from a stranger, a hug from your child, or a look from your spouse. Be grateful for living in a place where you can define yourself as you choose, where you enjoy the freedom to become your best self. Be grateful for the blue sky, the white clouds, the flowers, or the green grass. Heck, be grateful for your heart beating and never having to think about it.

Again, success without fulfillment and happiness is a massive failure. So I encourage you today to find gratitude in the small things and let your gratitude grow from there. When you can train yourself to be grateful for a simple lunch or for a hug, then these little things add up, and you become more meaningfully grateful daily.

Happiness Habit #9: Don't Settle For Good Enough

Don't settle for things being just okay. This acceptance will take away your happiness in a flash. Don't say things like, "My relationship is good enough." Instead, say, "My relationship might not be perfect, but I'm going to work hard at making it better." Strive for greatness in every part of your life. When you settle for just okay, whether it relates to income, a job, or a relationship, you lose out on much of the joy life has to offer.

Say no to just being okay. Get that terminology out of your life because subconsciously, that means you're telling yourself, "You're not good enough. You don't deserve better. Other people get to be happy and get to live abundantly, but you don't. It's good enough for just where you are." The heck with that! Stop telling yourself things are okay because you're subconsciously ruining your chances for happiness and for the joy and fulfillment that lie beyond.

You don't have to say, "My life is perfect right now." You could just be honest and say, "It is okay today, but I'm going for more, so keep going! Just okay is not good enough. There is a next-level life, and it's your turn to grab it.

Happiness Habit #10: Be Part of Something Bigger

This habit delves into the profound aspect of seeking spiritual connection or cultivating a relationship with a higher power. It's about transcending the confines of individual existence and immersing oneself in the vastness of something greater. By embracing this principle, you open yourself to a realm of spiritual growth and fulfillment that extends beyond the boundaries of your own perception.

Allowing yourself to become a part of something larger than life itself is transformative. It's a journey of exploration and discovery, where you delve into various avenues of spirituality that resonate with your innermost beliefs and convictions. Whether you find solace in general spirituality, the teachings of Zen Buddhism, the structure of organized religion, or foster a deeply personal relationship with the divine, the key lies in embracing what speaks to your soul.

When you align yourself with a higher purpose or a spiritual path, you tap into a wellspring of profound wisdom, guidance, and grace. This connection elevates your consciousness, infusing your life with meaning, purpose, and a profound sense of interconnectedness with all existence. Through this bond, you transcend the limitations of ego and individual identity, experiencing a profound sense of unity with the universe.

In essence, by immersing yourself in something greater than yourself, you unlock the door to boundless joy, peace, and fulfillment. It's a journey that leads you to the core of your being, where you discover the true essence of happiness—a radiant light that emanates from within and illuminates the path toward spiritual enlightenment.

CHAPTER 8:
THE QUICK HACKS TO SUCCESS

Take Creative Time Daily

We often fall into routines, living the same schedule day after day. It can feel like we're stuck on a hamster wheel, just spinning our wheels without progress. When this happens, our creativity, new ideas, dreams, visions, and inventions struggle to flourish.

Allocate ten to thirty minutes each day to simply think creatively. Don't respond to emails, review your to-do list, text, or browse social media. Just think. Personally, I do this after my morning workout and before my kids wake up. I focus on what's next for my life: What should I convey in my books? What new idea can I share with people today that will have the most transformative impact? What's my next TV show going to be?

As you give yourself permission to exercise your creativity, you'll find the creative juices start flowing. Don't underestimate your creativity; you possess it. Like most people, you might not give yourself credit for all your innovations. Perhaps you've invented a new relationship, a business, a career, or a character that brings laughter to your spouse. Nothing in life comes to us unless we first conceive it. Look around you: that lamp, that chair, that painting—someone envisioned them first, and then they became reality. Forgetting to take creative time every day deprives a part of your soul, and you don't want it to wither. Sometimes, I dedicate an entire day solely to being creative, exploring things that stimulate my mind and ignite my passion, keeping me eager for the next level of life.

Everyone has their own definition of creative time. It could involve painting, writing, sculpting, inventing, digital design, or countless other activities that spark your creativity. Whatever it may be, schedule the time and make it a daily practice.

Observe Other Jobs For Gratitude

What does that mean, exactly? I know we discussed gratitude earlier, but I want to offer you some additional insights into recognizing and expressing it. Whether you're acknowledging something significant or minor, it's important to find ways to manifest this feeling in the world. Yet, at times, this can be challenging, right? You're busy, juggling multiple tasks simultaneously, and gratitude isn't always at the forefront of your thoughts.

So, here's what I do: I observe other people's jobs to cultivate a sense of gratitude consciousness. Regardless of your profession, I understand it can be stressful. Moreover, it may feel overwhelming or leave you questioning the significance of your contributions. Thus, when I see individuals hard at work, getting their hands dirty, I silently extend my gratitude to them. I send thoughts of appreciation and acknowledgment their way.

Setting Gratitude Alarms

In today's world, where our cell phones serve as our personal assistants for almost every aspect of life (except perhaps using the bathroom for us), I've found it incredibly useful to leverage technology to cultivate gratitude. Amidst the whirlwind of our daily routines, it's all too easy to overlook opportunities to express gratitude. We can find ourselves caught up in frustration, overwhelm, annoyance, or even pessimism, losing sight of the simple joys that surround us.

That's why I've incorporated a simple yet powerful practice into my daily routine: setting gratitude alarms on my phone. At three different times each day, these alarms serve as gentle reminders to pause, reflect, and express gratitude.

At 3:00 PM, as the midday rush begins to settle in, a message pops up on my screen: "Be optimistic, enthusiastic, and loving." This reminder encourages me to infuse positivity into the remainder of my day, approaching tasks and interactions with a renewed sense of energy and kindness.

Later, as the day progresses and challenges may arise, another alarm goes off, bearing the message, "You can handle anything." This affirmation serves as a beacon of resilience, reminding me of my inner strength and ability to overcome obstacles with grace and determination.

Finally, at 7:00 PM, as the day draws to a close, the alarm chimes once more, gently nudging me to remember, "You are truly blessed." In these moments of reflection, I pause to acknowledge the abundance in my life, from the simplest pleasures to the most profound blessings.

These gratitude alarms provide me with precious opportunities to take a 30-second break from the hustle and bustle of daily life and reconnect with a sense of appreciation for everything I have. Moreover, they serve as powerful tools for shifting my mindset, helping to realign my perspective and cultivate a more positive outlook.

By incorporating these simple yet impactful reminders into my daily routine, I've discovered that gratitude becomes not just a fleeting sentiment, but a guiding force that shapes my interactions, my attitude, and ultimately, my experience of the world.

Stash Cash

You must make a habit of putting money away. I don't care if you make $500 a week or $500,000 a week; save some of it. There are certain people in the world, and maybe you know some, who will spend as much money as they make and more. If they make a dollar, they're going to spend $1.25.

But you've heard this advice before. Parents, financial advisors, and spouses may have all insisted that you start saving. This success hack, however, isn't as much about money as it is about confidence.

When you have money put away, it does something for your confidence. You will know in the back of your mind that you can weather any storm. If you have a bad month, a bad three months, break your leg, can't work, you can handle it. You possess peace of mind knowing that you and your family are going to be okay until you're back on your feet.

On the other hand, if you have no savings, you're always going to worry about your future, even if only subconsciously. And that is the worst feeling in the world. All it does is tug away at your confidence and peace of mind. You'll start thinking, "If I have another bad couple of months I won't be able to pay the rent. I have nothing saved for my retirement and I have nothing in savings. I have nothing to fall back on!" So I encourage you, no matter what your income, make a habit of stashing something away every single week of your life, even in the bad weeks. It's not about the money you're stashing away as much as it's about the feeling of confidence that helps you make better decisions moving forward.

Have you ever heard the phrase, "Scared money makes no money?" If you have no money stashed away, you're going to make decisions very cautiously, avoiding risk to feel safe. Because of this, you might miss out on taking an educated gamble that could lead to a big payoff. If you have no money stashed away, you're going to stay at that job you hate because you have no cushion. But if you stash money away for three or four years and your boss comes in and finally treats you so badly that you can't take it, you have the option to quit. But if there's no money, you'll swallow your pride and take the abuse. I don't care if you save $10 a week, $100 a week, or $1000 a week, whatever amount you can put away, do it. It will give you more than just a savings account.

Spoil Yourself Randomly

This might seem to contradict my previous point, but hear me out: you can save and spoil yourself. I don't have hundreds of cars and thousands of shoes because, to me, that's a waste. But I do indulge myself and my family with things that truly matter to us and from which we derive value.

For example, I know I spend three times as much as the average person on our household groceries because everything in my house is organic. I don't want my family eating food chock full of chemicals. Occasionally, I'll take the family on incredible trips, stay at the best places, and pamper ourselves. I love experiencing a great meal with the family, regardless of the cost. These are my rewards for my hard work, and they motivate me to strive for greater success. So when I say "spoil yourself," that's what I'm talking about. Treat yourself to things that evoke positive emotions, and if the spending creates lasting memories, even better.

If you stash cash and spend less on things that don't hold much meaning for you, when it's time to spoil yourself with things that truly matter, you'll have the means to do so. Spoiling yourself can give you glimpses of what could become the norm and push you to implement strategies and make decisions to better your life.

Invest in Yourself

I truly believe that we die when we stop learning. When it comes to life, we're either climbing or we're sliding. If you want to make more money in retirement, have more time for yourself, and enjoy more freedom, then never stop investing in yourself. Gaining more knowledge will transform your life experience into wisdom, and wisdom will provide you with the insight and guidance to reach your next level. Make sure you are learning from someone who has achieved what you aspire to on a grander scale. Get a mentor or a coach. Do an internship. Absorb knowledge from those who have walked the path to success you desire. Do you have someone to model yourself after or help keep you accountable?

Draw Energy From Your Frequent Smiles

I am optimistic, and I love people; it's as simple as that. But I know it can be a challenge to maintain this positive, friendly outlook. Sometimes we get so busy and caught up in our own worlds that we put our heads down and ignore people who we think don't matter because we're too busy to notice them. The delivery truck driver, the building custodian, and the restaurant server may go unnoticed. But then, someone with influence walks into the room, and only then do we put on our friendly faces. I promise you, I have never in my life treated a server badly. I'm always nice and polite, and I'm consciously aware to smile and make eye contact with everybody I interact with. This isn't just a decision to be "nice"; it's a choice to plug into the power source provided by an upbeat, human-centric attitude.

Now, you can't be "on" all the time. But you also don't want to be the person who treats somebody well because of what you think you can get out of them. Instead, wouldn't it be better to make an effort to appreciate everyone daily and give a quick smile as often as you can? Think about it, how much energy does that take? Not much at all, yet it will actually improve your state of mind and boost your energy while potentially making someone else's day.

Find The Good In The Bad

If you can create a habit of finding the good when things go wrong, your life will be transformed. So many people experience setbacks in their lives and then dwell on them for years. But along the road, someone might say, "You know, it's a good thing that relationship didn't work out because I found the love of my life," or "You know what, it was actually good that my first business failed because I learned from it, and that experience helped my next business succeed."

How many people do you know who avoid committing to relationships because they had their hearts broken years ago? Or do you know someone who won't start a new company because a business venture failed in the past? I believe that everything that happens in our lives happens for us, and there is a lesson and something good in all of it. If you can create a habit of finding that good sooner rather than later, you'll change your life.

Bounce Back Fast

I've been successful for many reasons, but my ability to bounce back from setbacks quickly is near the top of the list. Why not be the person among your peers, coworkers, or employees who rebounds from failure or overcomes obstacles faster than anyone else? I have self-programmed this habit or "hack" of fast rebounding, and it has paid huge dividends. How long do you linger on things when they go wrong? How long do you replay the situation over and over again in your mind? Learn from it, but pick up the pieces and move on with that experience in hand. The people who fail the fastest are the ones who find the solution the quickest.

Think Solution, Not Problem

It's unfortunate that when something goes wrong, people tend to obsess about why it happened, whose fault it was, and "why me?" Honestly, what good is that thinking in most cases? Yes, learn from it, but train your brain to be solution-oriented. Let's take the simplest example on the planet. What happens when a glass of milk spills? Yes, you can obsess and ask, how did that fall, who made it fall, will it stain the floor, will it smell, or think something along the lines of, "Why always me? I'm in a hurry and don't need this." But someone with a solution-oriented thought process would simply get a towel, clean up the spill, and get a new glass of milk. Use your energy wisely; learn from mistakes but then move on quickly with solutions.

Develop a habit that when things go wrong, you immediately ask, "How do I fix it? What steps can I take right now to lessen the damage?" Make a habit to focus all of your energy on the solution, not on dwelling on why it happened or who's to blame.

Ask Happy People

Every time I encounter individuals who are always smiling and seem to find joy in everything, I strike up a conversation with them. I'll ask, "What do you do to stay happy?" As you might have guessed by this point, I love asking people what brings them happiness. Sometimes, I receive a funny one-liner as a response, and I just chuckle and continue on my way. Other times, I'm fortunate to receive a thoughtful answer that leaves a lasting impact on me. When you encounter happy people, engage with them, and discover what they are doing to maintain that joyful demeanor.

My wonderful friend John laughs more than anyone I know. Despite owning and managing a multi-million dollar company, juggling numerous responsibilities and pressures, and raising three young children, he still finds the simplest things humorous, and his laughter is infectious. Naturally, I asked him what brings him happiness. He shared, "I personally reflect every day on how fortunate I am to have been born when I was, to live where I do, and to have the family I have." As you can see, there's nothing groundbreaking about John's approach. He doesn't possess a magic happiness button. Instead, he has found contentment through a routine of gratitude.

Go To Your Happy Place

I touched on this in the happiness habit chapter, but this success habit emphasizes focusing on one particular happy place or thought. Sometimes, we find ourselves in funks and need quick hacks to liberate ourselves from negative moods and realign our minds and souls. For me, my happy place is reminiscing about my childhood and spending time with my grandmother. Being with her felt like basking in a warm, comforting light, and her presence enveloped me in a sense of security. She taught me how to cook Italian food, and I'd spend hours with her on Sundays while she prepared the most delicious Italian dishes imaginable. Memories like those are my happy place. So when I'm feeling down, I retreat to them. I encourage you to find your own happy place and make it a habit that when you're having a rough day, you remind yourself to visualize this sanctuary. Once you lift yourself out of your funk, you'll find clarity of thought returning.

Live Long & Prosper

The signature phrase from Star Trek is worth applying to your life. If you don't have a healthy body, it's hard to have a healthy life and healthy thoughts. An Indian proverb says, "A healthy person has a thousand wishes but a sick person only has one." How true is that statement? This isn't a health book, and I don't claim to be an expert. But knowledge of healthy lifestyles is easier to find now than at any other time in history. Search it out and create habits that get you in optimal health. Why make all the money and attain all the fulfillment and abundance you desire if you can't be the parent, grandparent, leader, or spouse you know lives inside you?

To live long and prosper, you've got to exercise. It may be hard to start this habit, but once you make it a part of your life and you feel and see the benefits, you'll be hooked. You can find amazing workouts to fit your body and your fitness level online. Heck, you can hire a coach to keep you accountable and help you with a routine. But whatever you have to do, make it happen. I find that a few things keep me exercising. First, I want to be an example to my children. I want them to see me making exercise a part of my life and not treat it like a chore. I know this to be true: kids do what you do, not what you say. Also, I want to be an active dad and someday, an active grandparent. I'm sure you want the same.

Here are a few other ways to make exercise a habit. First, create a fitness challenge with a friend, whether it's weight loss, pants size, a 5k, or a before-and-after picture contest. A challenge makes it more likely you'll get engaged with the program and stay there. Next, I recommend mixing it up! Don't do the same thing every day! Go for a walk, run, ski, swim, bike, do some weights, row a boat, play tennis, or do short sprints. Just get in the habit of doing something different daily. When you exercise, you do everything better. You make wiser food choices, you refrain from adult beverages more often, and you even start to sleep better. On top of that, you start looking better. It's truly addicting! So, why not start today?

Take Time To Understand

When someone does something to make you feel slighted, underappreciated, snubbed, or disrespected, you become upset. That's understandable. But many times, we don't truly understand how they feel, and we simply assume their negative intent. And as I mentioned previously, this can cause us to waste energy, thoughts, time, and focus. It happens sometimes without even knowing it, and we have to stay away from this energy and time grabber. We are so much better off not wasting our time on the perceived sense that someone is doing us wrong.

I had this happen with my daughter's friend's father. Every time I saw the guy, I felt he was snubbing me. I remember thinking, "Well, he must have a problem with me." He never smiled, barely said hi when I tried greeting him a few times. I convinced myself that he was snobbish or opinionated and foolishly never talked to him about this subject. Finally, one day, I just decided to sit down and chat with him. He and I talked, and I discovered that I was completely wrong about the guy! He was just shy and a little insecure. He turned out to be the furthest thing from pretentious: A humble guy and a great dad; he just lacked the confidence to communicate well with people he barely knew.

Forcing myself to understand a situation before I react has been transformational in my life. Make it a habit to pause in any circumstances that offend you, no matter how bad the offense may seem. So much energy and stress can be avoided if we try to understand why people are doing what they do; or if necessary, we can avoid this wasted energy by deciding it is not going to affect our mood, no matter what. If you find out your spouse lied to you, your children lied to you, somebody at work is trying to undermine you, somebody at the gym is making fun of you, or someone went behind your back, stop and take a breath. After any upsetting event that happens in your life, taking a breath and refusing to react in the moment can lower your stress. Make the effort to understand where that person is coming from. Look through their eyes and then respond. Letting yourself go down the rabbit hole of assumptions is one of the largest energy drainers there is. So make it a habit: Decide not to do it.

Don't Judge

Easier said than done, I know. But when people ask me about times in my life when the biggest shifts or changes happened, I always reflect back on the moment when I completely let go of judgments. Can anyone be perfect? No, of course not. But can you get pretty darn close? Heck, yeah! And the results are life-changing.

When we judge, we're literally expending energy, thoughts, and time on something that's none of our business, or that we often lack sufficient knowledge of to make a judgment. As a child, I grew up around people who were very judgmental, and I think some of that attitude seeped into my young adult attitudes, even though I would've considered myself a non-judging person. Then one day it hit me - I was making judgments about people, and I had no idea what kind of circumstances were causing them to act as they did.

Sometimes you might see overweight people, and as your default reaction, you assume they're lazy or just have no control when it comes to their eating. When you see alcoholics, you think they have no self-discipline and that they should just stop drinking. When you see individuals who are grumpy or disrespectful, you think they are bad people. These default mechanisms live inside all of us. But when you get rid of your judgments, a whole part of your soul opens up for new exploration and growth.

As you can see, I love sharing by example. And I want to make this point in my children's lives at a young age so they can be judgment-free their entire lives. For the last five Christmases, after the kids open their presents and we have our morning routine, we jump in the car and drive to downtown Phoenix, armed with bagged lunches that contain $100 bills. We drive street by street, alley by alley, to find homeless people on Christmas morning and hand each one of them a lunch bag. We then say "Merry Christmas," and as we pull away, in so many cases, they are crying or shocked or saying thank God and thank you. And it's about more than the food and the money. It's about having the chance to feel that someone cares.

And my children are old enough to realize that people will say, "Why are you giving money to the homeless? They should work, they're lazy, they have options, they will use it for drugs or alcohol." And maybe that's the case in some instances, but who are we to judge?

Rather than pulling away from someone who's barely dressed, completely dirty, or smells horrible, the lessons I'm able to share with my children are the ones I want to become permanent in their souls. I get to teach my children that we don't know if the homeless people's families threw them out, if they were molested, if they were beaten, if they have a severe learning disability that no one noticed. I share with my children that there are a million reasons the homeless could be where they are. Some may be on drugs, and may use alcohol, and maybe that's the only thing that quiets the noises in their heads. I can tell my kids that we have no idea why they are there, but we can wish them well, let them know someone cares, pray for them, and find gratitude for the blessings we've had in our lives.

Yes, this is a lesson for my children from a dad who had a tougher childhood than they are experiencing. And yes, I may be doing this to help create adults who have empathy, caring spirits, no judgment, and have gratitude. But at the same time, I continue to do things like this to cement those values into my own life and heart. So stop judging and watch your heart, your life, your mind, your world, and your income continue to open up.

Help Those Who Are Worse Off Than You

This may seem like the same advice that I offered in the previous habit, but bear with me and you'll see the difference here. A few years ago, a friend of mine introduced me to Joel Osteen and invited me to fly to Houston to attend a service. I remember being in awe of the size and beauty of the church, as well as the multitude of smiling, happy people in attendance. I had the privilege of sitting next to Joel's wife and mother and truly enjoyed the experience. I must confess, it was the first time I had been in church in quite some time.

As I listened to Joel share stories, one in particular resonated deeply with me. Although it's been a while, I'll share it as closely as I can recall. He said something along the lines of the following: "When you think things are really bad in your life, when you believe you don't have enough money, love, health, or joy, go help somebody who's much worse off than you are. When you think your relationship is bad, visit a place where battered women need help and donate your time or money. When you feel you deserved that raise and feel slighted, visit a homeless shelter. Our problems are our own, and they are significant, and we still feel the pain. But it is impossible to feel sad or depressed and grateful at the same time. Make it a habit to help those worse off than yourself, especially when you are feeling down. When you help others who are worse off, your gratitude will rise and push your stress away. It's a win for everyone."

Helping others isn't a totally selfless act. As important as it is to lend a hand to those in need for its own sake, realize that you're going to benefit too.

Do Your Best Always

I know so many people who hate what they do for a living; they are dreaming, hoping, and trying as hard as they can to find the career or business they know they will love. But until you find that thing you love to do, use this quick success hack: do the absolute best you can, even if you hate it, until your next level kicks in.

Yes, it doesn't matter what it is; always give it 110%. Remember my earlier story of billionaire John Paul DeJoria, who swept floors in places the boss couldn't even see, and it set a success habit he followed for the rest of his life? Even though you may not like a particular task or job, do it amazingly well, and the benefits and habits learned will be priceless. When I was in high school and during the few years following, I used to fix wrecked cars in a collision shop with my dad. It was dirty and smelly work that, on many days, gave me a headache from the chemicals. My nails were dirty, my clothes looked like crap, and the truth is I hated it. But you would have never known how I felt by how I carried myself. If anybody walked into that collision shop, I know they thought to themselves, "Damn, this guy loves his job!" What they saw was that I did that job to the best of my ability every day, and with a smile to boot.

My first real estate deal was made possible by someone who had often visited the collision shop. We would chat, laugh, and I think he really liked my enthusiasm. One day I told him my story about some real estate deals I was working on and how I was juggling money but still making it happen. He ended up lending me over $80,000 because he saw my enthusiasm. Would I have received that investment if he had walked in and I had a crappy, negative attitude? The guy wouldn't have given me the time of day! Yes, I hated fixing cars, but my habit was to do the absolute best that I could until I reached the next level of my life. This one instance was a shift in that direction. The real estate deal resulted in over $1,000,000 in sales. True story!

I love to share examples from my own life that reveal the power of the right success habits or "hacks," as they've become part of my routine. But I'm not the only one creating these hacks and habits; they are also the habits of the highest achieving, most successful people on the planet.

I met Josh Bezoni a little over 9 years ago in Hawaii at a weekend Mastermind. At that time, he was running a decent-sized company and doing fairly well in the nutrition space. We hit it off through the years. Then Josh hit hard times with his company, and it went out of business. I flew to meet him in Colorado about 6 years ago when this was happening, and I remember walking through his old office. It was like a ghost town, empty desks everywhere, and it was truly sad to see. I could feel that my friend was doing his best to put on a good face, but he was heartbroken.

A year or so later, Josh invited me to a small event he did in Austin, Texas. It was really his coming-out party in a sense. He had spent sufficient time trying to learn what went wrong, getting over the negative stories and self-doubt in his head, and he was ready to jump back into the entrepreneurial world, even though he literally had no money to start over.

Fast-forward from this moment of reinvention to today, and Josh is the founder and CEO of BioTrust Nutrition, one of the world's leading premium nutrition brands. His company does hundreds of millions of dollars in sales, employs many great people, and provides outstanding products, some of which I use daily. What happened? How did Josh go from failure and overwhelming stress of closing a business, with no seed money to start, to a dominating world brand? His answer was, "I discovered through my success and failures, through trial and error that I had to change and create new habits."

Over the years, he's been incredibly successful in many roles: entrepreneur, nutritionist, and philanthropist. So while I was writing this section of the book, I called Josh and asked if he would share his new habits or success hacks with us. Josh was excited to share the routines that changed everything for him and made a recording, immediately sending it to me. One of the key habits he shared was:

"Hire people who have already done what you want to do." Josh referred to this as his number one success habit and talked about how this is exactly what he did when he started BioTrust Nutrition. Most people think they can train people to do a job, but there's no substitute for experience—especially when they have it and you don't. Josh shared, "Don't hire great soldiers that you can train to be great in their positions, hire generals who know their roles better than you do and let them hire the soldier underneath them."

Delegate anything that's not your unique ability. Listen to Josh explain why this is such an important hack: "For 10 years, I was stuck in a company that I owned, and it was almost like a prison. I was doing all the work. … I had a very small team, and I was making good profits, but my life was completely miserable. I was working 80 hours a week. I could have easily taken some of the profits and delegated and hired more people, but I felt I had to do it all or it wouldn't get done right. When that original company closed and I had time to examine what went wrong and what could go right in the future, I knew this had to change. When I started Bio Trust, I came out of the gate delegating everything that wasn't my unique ability, and I watched the magic unfold in front of my eyes… I was a happier person, and I wasn't doing things that I didn't like… Accounting and HTML programming and all these things that I had tried to do in the past. When I focused on my unique abilities, which are hiring the right people, creating the big vision for the company, and putting the right teams together, I made the biggest impact possible and watched all areas of my business and personal life go to the next level."

Feed your daily motivation just like you feed your body. What Josh means by this is that you have to do something every day to remind yourself why you're doing what you're doing. Here's how Josh describes his application of this habit: "Sometimes I make my own inspirational thought leaders. Every day I feed positive energy and positive information into my brain and remind myself what my goals are... Life can get hard sometimes, none of us are immune to that, no matter what level of success you are currently achieving. So we can decide to focus on what's not going right, or we can get daily motivation from any source possible and get our thoughts focused on a better version of ourselves. If you are going to think, it may as well be about why you want more and the positive thoughts about how you will get there."

From afar, I was a witness to how Josh's changing habits allowed him to not only rebound but to create a business and a life that is truly inspirational. Josh made mistakes, felt he let others down, believed he wasn't good enough. Is that unlike any feelings you and I have had or are having right now? No, of course not, because we are all so similar. Yet some people choose to stay in that place of despair, to keep the same routines and repeat the same patterns day after day, year after year. Unfortunately, life doesn't one day become amazing by accident. You have to decide it is going to be amazing. Josh is a shining example of someone who knew what he wanted, learned from his mistakes instead of wallowing in them, shifted his habits, and achieved greatness.

Focus with passion on one thing, and only one thing. This is a hack I believe in with all my heart, and I think you will too when you "hear" Josh describe it: I'm kind of ADD, and so I'd start a hundred businesses if I could. So I have rules in place where I can only have one thing, and I can tell if it is running by itself and is a success. I don't move on to something else, so it's forced focus (my term for this approach) because entrepreneurs will go all over the place and have a hundred projects, and none of them really take off. "So, it's a hard discipline but you have to force-focus."

Use Josh's success hacks, the ones I've listed, or modify and create some of your own. These small but impactful habits or hacks can be incorporated into your life starting right now. And, like I said earlier, it's about replacing current habits that simply are not empowering your future. If we work on our habits one day at a time, then life will never be the same again.

CHAPTER 9: HAVE AN ABUNDANT MINDSET

God's dream for your life is that you would be abundantly blessed so that you can generously bless others. As David beautifully expressed, "My cup runs over." God is an overflow God, but here's the key: you can't harbor thoughts of lack, scarcity, and struggle and expect to experience abundance. If you've been under prolonged pressure and struggling to make ends meet, it's understandable to develop a limited mindset. You might find yourself thinking, "I'll never escape this neighborhood," or "I'll never have enough to send my kids to college." While you may be in that situation now, it doesn't mean you have to remain there.

God is known as El Shaddai, the God of More than Enough. He's not the God of Barely Enough or the God of Just Help Me Make It Through. He's the God of Overflow, the God of Abundance. Psalm 35 encourages us to continually proclaim, "Let the Lord be magnified who takes pleasure in the prosperity of His children." This declaration was intended to cultivate an abundant mindset among His people. Your life tends to move in the direction of your predominant thoughts. Therefore, if you constantly dwell on thoughts of lack, scarcity, and struggle, you'll find yourself gravitating towards those very things.

Throughout the day, immerse yourself in thoughts of overflow, abundance, and the knowledge that God takes pleasure in prospering you. Allow these affirmations to shape your mindset and guide your actions, knowing that as you focus on abundance, you open yourself up to experience the fullness of God's blessings in your life.

BARELY ENOUGH, JUST ENOUGH AND MORE THAN ENOUGH

In the scripture, the Israelites had been in slavery for many years. That was the land of Barely Enough. They were just enduring, surviving, barely making it through. One day God brought them out of slavery and took them into the desert. That was the land of Just Enough. Their needs were supplied, but nothing extra. It says their clothes didn't wear for forty years. I'm sure they were grateful. I don't particularly want to wear these same clothes for the next forty years. If I have to, I'm not going to complain, but that's not my idea of abundance. It wasn't God either. God eventually took them into the Promised Land. That was the land of More Than Enough. The food and supplies were plenteous. The bundles of grapes were so large that two grown men had to carry them. It's called "the land flowing with milk and honey". Flowing means it didn't stop. It never ran out. It continued to have an abundance. That's where God is taking you.

You may be in the land of Barely Enough right now. You don't know how you're going to make it through next week. Don't worry. God hasn't forgotten about you. God clothes the lilies of the field. He feeds the birds of the air. He is going to take care of you.

You may be in the land of Just Enough. Your needs are supplied. You're grateful, but there's nothing extra, nothing to accomplish your dreams. God is saying, "I didn't breathe My life into you to live in the land of Barely Enough". Those are seasons. Those are tests. But they are not permanent. Don't put your stakes down. You are passing through. It is only temporary. God has a Promised Land for you. He has a place of abundance, of more than enough, where it's flowing with provision, not just one time, but you'll continue to increase. You will continue to have plenty.

If you're in the land of Barely Enough, don't you dare settle there. That is where you are; it is not who you are. That is the location; it's not your identity. You are a child of the Most High God. No matter what it looks like, have this abundant mindset. Keep reminding yourself, "God takes pleasure in prospering me. I am the head and never the tail".

The scripture says God will supply our needs "according to His riches". So often we look at our situation and think, I'll never get ahead. Business is slow, or I'm in the projects. I'll never get out. But it's not according to what you have; it's according to what He has. The good news is God owns it all. One touch of God's favor can blast you out of Barely Enough and put you into More Than Enough. God has ways to increase you beyond your normal income, beyond your salary, beyond what's predictable. Quit telling yourself, "This is all I'll ever have. Granddaddy was broke. Momma and Daddy didn't have anything. My dog is on welfare. My cat is homeless." Let go of all that and have an abundant mentality. "This is not where I'm staying. I am blessed. I am prosperous. I am headed to overflow, to the land of More Than Enough".

SKINNY GOAT OR FATTED CALF

I received a letter from a young couple. They had both been raised in low-income housing. All they saw modeled growing up was lack, struggle, can't get ahead. Their families had accepted it, but not this couple. They had been coming to Lakewood and didn't have a not enough mentality. They knew God had a Promised Land in store for them. They took a step of faith. On very average incomes, they decided to build their own house. They didn't take out a loan. Whenever they had extra funds, they would buy the materials and hire the contractors. A couple of years later, they moved into a beautiful house in a nice neighborhood, all debt-free. It was as though God had multiplied their funds. Not long ago they sold that house for twice what they had put into it. The lady wrote, "We never dreamed we would be blessed like today." She went on to say, "My grandparents always told me that if I had beans and rice that was good enough. But I always knew one day I would have steak."

"If you're going to become everything God has created you to be, you have to make up your mind as she did. You are not going to settle for beans and rice. You are not going to get stuck in the land of Just Enough, but you're going to keep praying, believing, expecting, hoping, dreaming, working, and being faithful until you make it all the way into the land of More Than Enough. Now, there is nothing wrong with beans and rice. Nothing wrong with surviving. But God wants you to go further. God wants you to set a new standard for your family. He is an overflow God, a more-than-enough God.

Jesus told a parable about a prodigal son. This young man left home and blew all of his money, wasted his inheritance, and decided to return home. When his father represents God, he said to the staff, "Go kill the fatted calf. We're going to have a party." But the older brother got upset. He said, "Dad, I've been with you this whole time, and you've never given me a skinny goat."

Let me ask you. Do you have a fatted-calf mentality, or do you have a skinny-goat mentality? Do you think beans and rice are good enough, or do you say, "I want some enchiladas. I want some fajitas. I want some sopaipillas"? You can live on bread and water. You can survive in the land of Barely Enough. We can endure the land of Just Enough. "Just Enough to make it through. Just enough to pay my bills this week." But that is not God's best. Your heavenly Father, the One who breathed life into you, is saying, "I have a fatted calf for you. I have a place for you in the land of More Than Enough."

Now don't go around thinking that you'll never get ahead. You'll never live in a nice place. You'll never have enough to accomplish your dreams. Get rid of that skinny-goat mentality and start having a fatted-calf mentality. God wants you to overflow with His goodness. He has ways to increase you that you've never dreamed.

One Touch of God's Favor

I received a letter from a single mother. She immigrated to the United States from Europe many years ago. English is not her first language. She had three small children and didn't know how she would ever be able to send them to college. It seemed as though she was at a disadvantage, living in a foreign country all alone, not knowing anybody.

She applied for a job as a secretary at a prestigious university. Several dozen other people applied for the same position. When she saw all the competition, she was tempted to feel intimidated. Negative thoughts were bombarding her mind. To make matters worse, the lady conducting the interview was harsh and condescending. But this mother didn't get frustrated. She didn't have an underdog mentality thinking, "What's the use? I'm at a disadvantage. I'll never get ahead." She had a fatted-calf mentality. She didn't see a way, but she knew God had a way.

All the applicants had to take a five-minute typing test. She was not a fast typist, but she started typing, doing her best. The bell went off signaling that her five minutes were up, so she stopped typing. But the lady in charge had gotten distracted answering a phone call and said to her gruffly, "Keep typing! That's not your bell." But it was her bell. It was right in front of her. She said, "Okay," and typed another five minutes. They added up the number of words she typed - ten minutes' worth - and divided it by five, and by far she had the best typing skills and ended up getting the job. One of the benefits of working for this university is that your children get to go to school for free. That was over thirty years ago. Today, all of her children have graduated from this very prestigious university, receiving over seven hundred thousand dollars in education free of charge.

One touch of God's favor can thrust you into more than enough. Don't talk yourself out of it. All through the day, say, "I am prosperous. I am coming into overflow. I will lend and not borrow."

A Place of ABUNDANCE

When the Israelites were in the desert in the land of Just Enough, they got tired of eating the same thing every day. They said, "Moses, we want some meat to eat out here." They were complaining, but at least for a little while, they had a fatted-calf mentality.

Moses thought, "That's impossible. Meat out here in the desert? Steak for two million people? There were no grocery stores, no warehouses to buy truckloads of meat." But God has ways to increase you that you've never thought of. God simply shifted the direction of the wind and caused a huge flock of quail to come into the camp. They didn't have to go after it. The food came to them. What's interesting is that quail don't normally travel that far away from the water. If there had not been a strong wind, the quail would have never made its way out there in the desert. What am I saying? God knows how to get your provision to you.

A statistician ran some numbers. Based on the size of the camp, the number of people, and enough quail to be three feet off the ground as the Scripture says, he concluded that there were approximately 105 million quail that came into the camp. That's an abundant God. He could have given them a couple of quail per person, which would have been four or five million quail. But God doesn't just want to meet your needs; He wants to do it in abundance. The question is, are you thinking skinny goat or are you thinking fatted calf?

"Well, Joe. I could never afford a nice place to live." Can I say this respectfully? Skinny goat. "I could never build that orphanage. I could never support other families. I can barely support my own family." Friend, God has a fatted calf, a place of abundance for you.

He is not limited by your circumstances, by how you were raised, or by what you don't have. He is limited by what you believe. Maybe you've had a skinny goat with you for years and years. You've become best friends. You need to announce to him today, "I'm sorry, but our relationship is over. It's done. We're going to be parting ways." He may cry and complain, "Baa-ah." He may ask, "Is there someone else?" Tell him, "Yes, I've found a fatted calf. No more thinking not enough, barely enough, just enough. From now on I'm thinking more than enough; an abundant mindset."

Pressed Down and Running Over

When you live with this attitude, God will bless you in ways you've never imagined. I talked to a lady who has been through a lot of struggles. For years she was barely making it, but every Sunday she and her two sons would be at Lakewood. In spite of all the obstacles, they didn't have a skinny-goat mentality. They were in the land of Barely Enough, but they didn't put their stakes down. They knew that wasn't their permanent address.

As a mother, you have to be faithful in the wilderness if you're going to make it into the Promised Land. I'm not saying that everything is going to change overnight. There are going to be seasons of testing and proving. Thoughts are going to tell you, "It's never going to change," but don't believe those lies. Keep being faithful right where you are, honoring God, thanking Him that you're coming into overflow.

This lady's son, from the time he was a little boy, always said that he was going to get a scholarship to go to college. He could have thought, "We're poor. I'm at a disadvantage." But his mother taught her sons that God is a God of abundance. A while back, her son graduated number two in his high school. He received not one scholarship, not two, not seven. He was awarded nine scholarships, totaling more than 1.3 million dollars! His undergraduate, his master's, and his doctorate degrees are paid for at Georgetown University. That's what happens when you say goodbye to the skinny goat and hello to the fatted calf.

Jesus talked about how when we give, it will be given back to us as good measure, pressed down, shaken together, and running over. What does that mean, pressed down? I used to make chocolate chip cookies with our children. The recipe calls for three-fourths of a cup of brown sugar. When you pour the brown sugar in, it's so thick and dense, even when it hits the mark for three-fourths, you have to press it down. When you do, you can put in about twice what it looked like initially.

That's what God is saying. When you look full, you think you're blessed and healthy. All you need is one scholarship. You just want the house to sell for what you put into it. You just want quail for a day or two. God says, "That's fine, but I am an overflow God. I'm more than enough God. I'm about to press down and make room for more of my increase. I'm going to press it down and show you my favor in a new way."

After He presses it down, He is going to shake it together and not just fill it to the top. He is going to take it one step further and give you so much that you're running over. You just wanted one scholarship. God says, "That's fine. I'm going to give you nine to make sure you're covered." You just wanted to get money out of the house. God says, "I'm going to cause it to sell for double." You just wanted quail for a day or two. God says, "I'm going to give you steak for a whole month." That's the way our God is. Why don't you get in agreement and say, "God, I'm ready. I'm a giver. I have an abundant mentality. Lord, I want to thank you for good measure, pressed down, shaken together, and running over in my life."

Out of Lack, Into a Good & Spacious Land

A friend of mine has a son who got his driver's license back and really wanted a car. His father said to him, "Let's believe that God will give you a car." Then the son replied, "Dad, God is not going to give me a car. You can buy me a car." He said, "No, let's pray." They asked God to somehow make a way that he could have a car. A couple of months later, this man's employer called him in and said, "For the last two years, we've made a mistake on your paycheck. We've been underpaying you." They handed him a check for five hundred dollars more than the car they had been hoping to buy.

The scripture says, "Is there anything too hard for the Lord?" There is no telling what God will do if you'll get rid of the skinny-goat mentality. God is about to press some things down. He is about to make room to show you His increase in a new way.

It says in the book of Exodus, "I am bringing you out of lack into a good and spacious land." Not a small land. Not a little place. Tight. Crowded. Not enough room. Receive this into your spirit. God is bringing you into a spacious land. A land of more than enough. A land of plenty of room. A land that's flowing with increase, flowing with good breaks, flowing with opportunity, where you not only have enough for yourself, but you're running over the space. Running over with supplies. Running over with opportunity. If you're not in a good and spacious place, my challenge is, don't settle there. Don't let the skinny-goat mentality take root. Don't think beans and rice are good enough. That is not your permanent address. It's only temporary. God is taking you to a good and spacious land.

"Well, Joel," you say, "are you one of those prosperity ministers?"

I don't like that term. That's somebody who talks only about finances. Prosperity to me is having your health. It's having peace in your mind. It's being able to sleep at night. Having good relationships. There are many things that money cannot buy. While I don't like the term prosperity minister, I can't find a single verse in the scripture that suggests we are supposed to drag around not having enough, not able to afford what we want, living off the leftovers, in the land of Not Enough. We were created to be the head and not the tail. Jesus came that we might live an abundant life. We represent Almighty God here on this earth. We should be examples of His goodness—so blessed, so prosperous, so generous, so full of joy—that other people want what we have.

If I brought my two children into your house and their clothes were all raggedly and worn out, with holes in their shoes, and their hair not combed, you would look at me and think, "What kind of father is he?" It would be a poor reflection on me. When you look good, dress well, live in a nice place, excel in your career, and are generous with others, that brings a smile to God's face. It brings Him pleasure to prosper you.

The Power To Get Wealth

My father was raised during the Great Depression. He grew up extremely poor and developed a poverty mindset. He was taught in seminary that you had to be poor to show God that you were holy. The church he pastored made sure he stayed holy by keeping him poor. He was making a little over one hundred dollars a week, trying to raise his children, barely surviving. One time he and my mom kept a guest minister in their home. Sunday after service, a businessman came up to my father and handed him a check for a thousand dollars. That's like five thousand dollars today. He said, "I want you to have this personally to help take care of the expenses of the guest minister." My father took the check by its corner as though it was contaminated. He said, "Oh, no, I could never receive this. We must put it in the church offering." He walked toward the offering plate, and with every step something said, "Don't do it. Receive God's blessing. Receive God's favor." He ignored it and dropped it in the offering plate. When he did, he said he felt sick to his stomach.

There is something inside us that says we're supposed to be blessed. We're supposed to live an abundant life. It's because we are children of the King. It was put there by our Creator. But here's the key: You have to give God permission to prosper you. You can't go around with a lack mentality, thinking, "I'll just take the leftovers to show everyone how humble I am. After all, God wouldn't want me to have too much. That would be greedy. That would be selfish." Get rid of that false sense of humility. That's going to keep you from an abundant life.

Consider these words from Deuteronomy 28 in The Message translation: God will lavish you with good things. He will throw open the doors of his sky vaults and rain down favor. You will always be top dog and never the bottom dog. You need to start seeing yourself as the top dog, not living off the leftovers, not able to afford what you want, in the land of Not Enough. Come over to the land of More Than Enough. It starts in your thinking. Give God permission to increase you. Give him permission to lavish you with good things.

We think, "Is it wrong for me to want to live in a nice house or drive a nice car? Is it wrong to want funds to accomplish my dreams or want to leave an inheritance for my children?" God is saying, "It's not wrong. I take pleasure in prospering you." If it was wrong to have resources, abundance, and wealth, why would God have chosen to start the new covenant with Abraham? Abraham is called the father of our faith. The scripture says, "Abraham was extremely rich in livestock and in silver and in gold." He was the Bill Gates of his day. God could have chosen anyone, but He chose Abraham—a man extremely blessed.

David left billions of dollars for his son to build the temple, and yet David is called "a man after God's own heart." Get rid of the thinking that God wouldn't want me to have much. That wouldn't be right. That might not look good. It's just the opposite. When you look good, it makes God look good. When you're blessed, prosperous, and successful, it brings Him honor.

I realize that everything I have comes from God. Whether it is the suit that I'm wearing, my car, my house, or my resources, it's God's goodness. You don't have to apologize for what God has done in your life. Wear your blessings well.

The Scripture says, "It is the Lord who gives you power to get wealth." God wouldn't give you power to do something and then condemn you for doing it. There is nothing wrong with having money. The key is to not let the money have you. Don't let it become the focus of your life. Don't seek that provision. Seek the provider. Money is simply a tool to accomplish your destiny and to advance His Kingdom.

A Thousand Times More

Victoria and I have big dreams in our hearts. It's going to take millions of dollars to do what's on the inside. These are not just dreams for ourselves, for a bigger this or a bigger that, but dreams to build orphanages and medical clinics. I can't do that with a limited, lacking, "God doesn't want me to have much" mentality. I realize that my Father owns it all. He makes streets out of gold. You are not going to bankrupt heaven by believing for an abundant life. All God has to do is go pick up a chunk of pavement and give it to you. When you have this abundant mindset and a desire to advance the Kingdom, God will lavish you with good things. He will open up the doors of His sky vault so that you not only accomplish your dreams, but you can also be a blessing to the world.

My prayer for you is found in Deuteronomy 1:11. It says, "May the Lord of your fathers increase you a thousand times more than you are." Can you receive that into your spirit? A thousand times more income. Most of the time our thinking goes TILT! TILT! TILT! It's because we've been hanging out with the skinny goat too long. It's time to cut him loose. It's time to have a fatted-calf mentality. God is about to press some things down. He is about to make room for more of His increase. Now get up every morning and say, "Lord, I want to thank you that you are opening up Your sky vaults today, raining down favor, and lavishing me with good things. I am prosperous."

If you'll have this abundant mentality, I believe and declare you won't live in the land of Just Enough or the land of Barely Enough, but you're coming into the land of More Than Enough.

ABOUT THE AUTHOR

Introducing T. Riojas, an author whose latest book explores the transformative power of self-care, patience, and compassion. Through heartfelt storytelling, T. Riojas invites readers to embark on a journey of self-discovery and growth. With gentle wisdom and heartfelt prose, T. Riojas reminds us of the importance of nurturing ourselves and extending kindness to others. Join T. Riojas as they shares their insights on cultivating patience, fostering compassion, and embracing the beauty of self-care in our daily lives.